Slim
for
Life

The Ultimate Health and Detox Plan

Dr. Gillian McKeith

Ⓟ

A PLUME BOOK

PLUME

Published by Penguin Group

Penguin Group (USA) Inc., 375 Hudson Street, New York, New York 10014, U.S.A.

Penguin Group (Canada), 90 Eglinton Avenue East, Suite 700, Toronto, Ontario, Canada M4P 2Y3 (a division of Pearson Penguin Canada Inc.)

Penguin Books Ltd., 80 Strand, London WC2R 0RL, England

Penguin Ireland, 25 St. Stephen's Green, Dublin 2, Ireland (a division of Penguin Books Ltd.)

Penguin Group (Australia), 250 Camberwell Road, Camberwell, Victoria 3124, Australia (a division of Pearson Australia Group Pty. Ltd.)

Penguin Books India Pvt. Ltd., 11 Community Centre, Panchsheel Park, New Delhi – 110 017, India

Penguin Group (NZ), 67 Apollo Drive, Rosedale, North Shore 0632, New Zealand (a division of Pearson New Zealand Ltd.)

Penguin Books (South Africa) (Pty.) Ltd., 24 Sturdee Avenue, Rosebank, Johannesburg 2196, South Africa

Penguin Books Ltd., Registered Offices: 80 Strand, London WC2R 0RL, England

Published by Plume, a member of Penguin Group (USA) Inc. Originally published in Great Britain by Penguin Books Ltd.

First American Printing, January 2008

10 9 8 7 6 5 4 3

Text copyright © Gillian McKeith, 2006
Portrait photography copyright © Colin Bell, 2006
Food photography copyright © Benoît Audureau, 2006

CIP data is available.
ISBN 978-0-452-28925-3

Printed in the United States of America
Set in New Clarendon and Trade Gothic

PUBLISHER'S NOTE

Neither the publisher nor the author is engaged in rendering professional advice or services to the individual reader. The ideas, procedures, and suggestions contained in this book are not intended as a substitute for consulting with your physician. All matters regarding your health require medical supervision. Neither the author nor the publisher shall be liable or responsible for any loss or damage allegedly arising from any information or suggestion in this book.

CONTENTS

INTRODUCTION

DAY 1: GOING TO NEW HEIGHTS OF ULTIMATE HEALTH

This is the book that will take you to new heights of wellness and new degrees of health on all levels: physically, emotionally, and spiritually. We go deeper and further than I have ever done before in any other book. For that to happen I want you to know where I'm coming from. I want you to feel you know me, and more importantly I want you to know yourself better. The following pages are the culmination of years of working with clients, distilled and ready for you to put straight into practice.

To succeed, you will find out how to really look at yourself on all levels: your diet, your lifestyle, your attitude, and your emotions. I will share with you some of the very same tools that I use with my clients. This book is a real workbook for you—in essence it's your own consultation.

Before we start, here's a story which just about sums me up! Anyone who knows me knows I am a bit wild about my mango smoothies. I just love them because they're so good for you, I can load them up with superfoods, minerals, and vitamins, and they taste so delicious. I start every day with a smoothie.

My brother tells me I'm obsessed, but I just say that I'm passionate about smoothies and your health. It's not that I'm obsessed, but I do now know that achieving ultimate health requires active engagement, passion, and determination. We control more about our own health than most people realize. But back to my Smoothie Story . . .

Several years ago, I was asked to be the keynote speaker to a convention of health practitioners and doctors in Sofia, Bulgaria. To prepare myself for the trip, I spent the night before my departure whipping up five separate flasks of mango smoothies. Upon arrival at the extremely nice hotel room in Sofia, I grabbed a smoothie flask. As I made the final twist of the lid, I vaguely felt some kind of a pressure build-up inside the flask. I was just looking forward to my smoothie, but then there was a loud pop as the lid disengaged itself and flew off like a rocket. I have never seen anything quite like it and probably never will again. A thick concoction of four finely blended ripe mangoes, three large bananas, and two peaches had exploded all over my hotel room:

the ceiling, the walls, the drapes, the beddings, and my clothes were all splattered and covered with mango goo.

I was horrified. You hear this kind of thing about British rock stars or an American heavy metal band trashing their hotel room. But whoever heard of a TV nutritionist from Scotland destroying the place with mango pudding? And then it dawned on me. I looked within myself and realized that any person who would travel almost 2,000 miles from home with five flasks of mango smoothies in tow must be a seriously passionate and determined nutritionist who will go to the end of the earth for ultimate health.

I don't want you to follow in my mango-exploding footsteps, but this is the kind of determination and passion for health that I want you to embrace. It is already within your grasp; you just need to learn how to unlock it. I will give you the tools to discover your own desires, set your goals, and achieve them. This book is like the roadmap; once you know the route, then the rest is easy. Flick the switch and discover the power to eat well, feel well, and look fab.

This book shows you the way to manifest a new you, a new body, new foods, new cells, a new attitude, and a renewed love and appreciation for yourself, so that your natural energy is free and clear to create ultimate health and happiness. And by the way, if you ever get the wild desire to travel halfway across the world with flasks of pressurized, nutrient-infused fruit smoothies ready for an imminent explosion, then just go for it and laugh your head off afterwards.

Wishing you Love & Light,

Gillian

Dr. Gillian McKeith (PhD)
www.drgillianmckeith.com
JANUARY 2006

level one
the wake-up call

THE FOOD DIARY

Many people convince themselves that they eat a healthy diet, when the reality is somewhat different. If you think you eat really well, see if this typical exchange between a new client and myself rings any bells. Here's how the play goes:

Gillian: Hi, nice to meet you.
Client: Hello, it's great to be here.
Gillian: Let's talk about your food. Do you eat well?
Client: Pretty well.
Gillian: And how do you feel?
Client: I'm bloated, tired, and I just don't seem to have much energy. I get jittery, suffer from headaches, sweet cravings, mood swings, stress, and insomnia. I just don't feel very healthy.
Gillian: Well, how would you evaluate your food intake?
Client: I think it's okay. Like everybody, I have my blips now and again.
Gillian: Give me an example of a blip.
Client: I like chocolate now and again.
Gillian: How much chocolate?
Client: Just a little piece of chocolate each day.
Gillian: Let's cut to the chase here. Be straight with me. I need to know, how many *bars* of chocolate are you eating each day?
Client: On average two, unless I feel really ratty, then it might be more, especially during my period.
Gillian: Please may I see your Food Diary?
Client: Fine. But it's not been a typical week. I really don't eat that much chocolate. This week was an exception. Really!

I look at the Food Diary, and I am shocked by the sheer number of chocolate bars that this woman is eating on a regular, daily basis. No wonder she's suffering. But she's taken the all-important first step toward making a positive change, and she'll soon know how good it feels to leave those headaches and cravings behind.

My point here is to illustrate that many people, when they meet me for the first time, tell me that they eat a good, healthy diet. Most think or say they eat healthy foods, almost like a trained, autopilot response. In reality though, when I start to delve further I often find that it is not so healthy after all, and then I get to the honest truth. There is often very little correlation between the first utterance of "I eat healthily" and the practical reality.

Seven-Day Diary

For the next seven days, I want you to get real, be honest with yourself, and write down in a notebook everything you eat and drink. And I mean *absolutely every morsel*. Do not exclude anything. This food and beverage diary exercise will help you make conscious rather than automated choices about the food you eat. Most unhealthy eating is a mindless, habitual, conditioned reaction to a wide variety of cues, few of which have to do with hunger. By writing down what you're doing, when you're doing it, and how you're feeling at the time, you will give yourself the opportunity to transform a habit into a conscious choice. It will help you to identify your goals and how you're going to achieve them.

A complete picture of you and your diet will open a window and give you an understanding of your eating habits and their effect on your life, energy levels, weight, and health. So, from the minute you get up until the minute you go to bed, I want you to document everything. It may seem like a pain at first, but once you get going you will soon get into the swing.

No Half-Measures

No half-measures here now. If you have a bar of chocolate every night, write that down. Excluding the chocolate from the list does not mean that you did not eat it! Include times of eating and drinking, quantities, brand names, and how the food is prepared—fried, steamed, grilled, baked—and whether or not the food is made from scratch, is fresh, packaged, microwaved, or raw/not cooked. Be as specific as possible, so even include the amount of sugar you add to tea, whether or not the tea is herbal or regular, if you add salt to your cooking, the amount of water you drink, and whether it is sparkling or still. The more detail, the more complete the picture of you.

Exercise

I also want you to take note of all the exercise you take, from walking to work to a full gym workout. Note down the time, what type of exercise, and how long.

Sleep

Keep a note of your sleep patterns. What time do you go to bed? How long does it take to fall asleep and how many unbroken hours of sleep do you have? Do you wake up energized or exhausted?

Food and Mood

Last but not least, note how you feel before eating a meal, a snack, any food or drink. You may feel energized, tired, restless, or just fine. Write down how you feel afterwards, *only* if you notice a difference. You may not experience any change and that is okay. Your feeling may be positive or negative. Write it down. Here are some guidelines to help:

1. How hungry do you feel before food? Are you hungry after food?
2. How do you feel physically? For example, do you feel headachy, shaky, or tired? If you feel just fine, do not make any comment.
3. How do you feel emotionally? For example, do you feel stressed, bored, apathetic, or happy? Are you upset about something while eating? Did you have an argument with someone before eating?
4. Observe how you feel afterwards, if you notice a change. Are you satisfied or still hungry? Are there any emotional feelings or physical changes? Are you sleepy, tired, energized? Don't go looking for something that is not there. Simply take note if you notice a physical feeling or emotion.

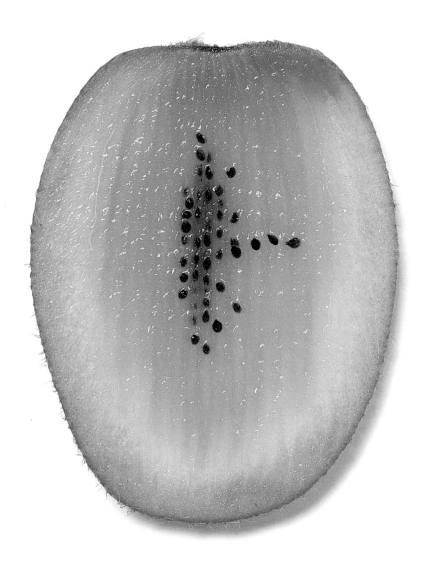

Dr. Gillian McKeith's dietary intake form

I promise to be 100 percent honest, truthful, and exact about everything I eat and drink over the next seven days.

Signature ....

1. Time of day
2. Food and beverage intake in detail, including quantities and brands if appropriate
3. How the food is prepared
4. Where and with whom the food is eaten
5. Moods/emotions

EXAMPLE DAY

Friday

7:00 a.m. Cup of tea. Slept badly, dreamt I was late for everything. Feel tired.

8:00 a.m. Hazelnut yogurt, 3½ oz., made with added cream and sugar.

10:00 a.m. Bottle of water.

1:00 p.m. Chicken salad sandwich, no mayo. Small bag of salted potato chips. Apple.

1:30 p.m. Cup of tea.

3:00 p.m. Feel tired and fed up. Chocolate bar.

4:00 p.m. Glass of water and cup of peppermint tea.

7:00 p.m. Glass of wine with handful of olives.

8:00 p.m. Dinner: swordfish and veggies, followed by lemon tart with fresh raspberries . . . washed down with another 2 glasses of wine.

11:00 p.m. Cup of tea, then bed.

THE COLLECTOR

I had a client once who was an investment banker. A confessed workaholic, he labored all hours and rarely left his office. Breakfast, lunch, and even dinner were eaten at his desk while he was talking on the phone and doing the big deals. When he made an appointment with me, I asked him to bring the wrappers of everything he ate and drank for a week. When he arrived, he lugged into my office a huge garbage bag, bursting at the seams, packed with a week's worth of what he had scarfed.

As we looked through the wreckage it was clear he had not eaten anything real for that entire week. Tumbling onto my desk came wrapper after wrapper from chocolate bars, sweets, chewing gum, sugary drinks—dozens of them—and a few greasy take-out wrappers. He was living on sweets.

We both surveyed the mountain of paper and plastic. Mr. Banker blurted out, "I know this cannot be good for me, but I have no clue what to do about it. I am too damn busy."

Excuse number one had hit his lips. The excuse I hear all the time. Too busy for what? Too busy to eat? Too busy to care? Too busy to live?

It turned out that the banker had been told by his doctor that he was a walking time bomb, heading for type II diabetes. He was exhausted all the time, 40 pounds overweight, plagued with headaches, and making costly mistakes at work. This moment of realization was the first step in his transformation to wellness: the glaring recognition for the first time of the cocktail of nonfoods, chemicals, additives, and rubbish that he was forcing his body to exist on.

The Collector in You

In addition to your Food Diary I want you to become a packaging collector this week. Keep all the packaging from everything that you eat and drink, healthy or unhealthy, for seven days. Put it all in a large box or a bag.

So, if you have a microwaveable ready meal on Tuesday night, I want you to keep the packaging with the ingredients listing. The same goes for take-out; hold on to all the bags and cartons that come with it. If you use ingredients to make something fresh, make a note of where the ingredients come from. For example, if you eat three fresh carrots, write this information on a piece of paper and add it to the bag with all the bottles, packets, and so on. If the carrots were organic, mark that information down too. By the end of seven days you may have quite a collection.

Why Am I Collecting?

1. To get in touch with exactly what you put into your body
2. To learn to read food labels
3. To start evaluating what is in the food that you are eating
4. To see just how much fresh food you are consuming versus processed food

THE RECKONING

At the end of the seven days, I want you to sit down in front of all of your packaging and take a good look through. You might be surprised or even horrified. This is a brilliant visual exercise for waking up to the reality of your diet.

GET INTO LABELS

The food label is a reliable, accurate, user-friendly source of valuable nutritional information. What you learn from reading and comparing food labels will help you to avoid ingredients and additives that may not be good for you. Knowledge leads to empowerment and better choices.

How Do I Read the Ingredients List?

The ingredients are listed in descending order by weight and include any color additives, preservatives, nutrients, fats, or sugars that have been added. So if a packet of food has sugar as the first ingredient, then you know that the sugar content within that food is high.

What about Food Additives?

There are over 14,000 man-made chemicals added to our food supply today. Our bodies are not designed to break down and digest so many chemicals and food additives. Be aware of the types of chemicals and food additives you are consuming. Some additives in our food have been linked to a variety of health problems including headaches, fatigue, and allergies.

TOP 10 FOOD ADDITIVES TO AVOID

- ► Acesulfame-K
- ► Artificial colorings
- ► Aspartame
- ► BHA & BHT
- ► Caffeine
- ► Monosodium Glutamate (MSG)
- ► Nitrite and Nitrate
- ► Potassium Bromate
- ► Sulfites
- ► Tartrazine

If you need a dictionary to decipher the label, chances are you should not be eating that food.

Food Claims

Claims are sometimes made on food packaging such as "low in fat and cholesterol" or "fortified with iron." Here's a quick guide to some of the problems associated with these claims.

WHAT IS FORTIFIED?

Fortified means that a nutrient that is not naturally present in a food has been added. Natural foods contain an abundance of nutrients that are instantly recognizable to the human body and so easily digested. The thousands of nutrients and phytochemicals found in natural foods work in perfect harmony with each other. Fortified foods tend to contain isolated nutrients that have been shown to be commonly deficient in our diet. The problem is that the natural synergy of the nutrients is lost when they are taken separately like this.

Foods fortified with calcium are one example. The type of calcium used is often calcium carbonate, which is poorly utilized and can lead to a buildup of calcium deposits that can actually cause health problems. Calcium utilization is affected by magnesium, vitamin D, boron, fiber, and the ratio of other minerals to the calcium. All of these are likely to be out of balance if calcium is added to a food. It's not the way nature intended it.

WHAT IS ENRICHED?

Rice is a good example. Everybody tells me how much they love white rice. But the difference between brown rice and white rice is not just in color. The milling and polishing that converts brown rice into white rice destroys approximately two-thirds of the vitamin B3, 80 percent of the vitamin B1, 90 percent of the vitamin B6, plus half of the manganese, half of the phosphorus, 60 percent of the iron, and all of the dietary fiber and essential fatty acids. The resulting white rice is simply a refined starch that is largely bereft of its original health-boosting nutrients. You'll probably find that white rice has been "enriched" with vitamins B1, B3, and iron. But the form of these nutrients when added back into the processed rice is not the same as in the original unprocessed version, and at least 11 lost nutrients are not replaced at all.

Keep Them Low

On the nutrition label, the nutrients that most people eat too much of are listed first. It is a good idea to read the labels and choose foods that are low in the following:

- Salt
- Sugar
- Saturated fat

Salt

Salt is needed by the body to help cells take up nutrients and balance fluid levels, but it is needed in only tiny amounts. The recommended limit of salt is 6g per day. Salt is hidden in so many foods, even before you shake it on your food. Try to make sure you eat "no added salt" foods as much as possible and instead of adding salt when cooking, add flavor through dried and fresh herbs.

When reading nutrition labels also watch out for "sodium," as 1g of sodium is roughly equivalent to 2.5g salt. Table salt is 40 percent sodium, and I want you to cut out using table salt completely. Too much salt can raise your blood pressure, which in turn can lead to heart disease, stroke, or kidney problems.

Sugar Junkies

Sugars are a type of carbohydrate that occurs naturally in foods such as fruits. Added sugars are those that do not occur naturally in a food but are added during processing or preparation. Foods containing added sugars provide calories but may have few vitamins and minerals. Frequently consumed foods with added sugars include soft drinks, cakes, cookies, pies, ice cream, sweets, chocolate, many ready meals, and some canned foods. Consuming too many of these foods may cause weight gain or prevent you from eating more nutritious foods.

Because added sugars are not always called "sugar," it can be difficult to identify them in food. Following is a list of just some of the names for added sugars. If one of these names appears first or second in the ingredients list, the food is probably high in added sugar.

- Brown sugar
- Cane juice
- Corn sweetener
- Corn syrup
- Dextrose
- Fructose
- Glucose
- High-fructose
- Invert sugar
- Lactose
- Maltose
- Raw cane sugar
- Raw sugar
- Sucrose syrup

The Fat Problem

Some fats are very good for you; in fact they are essential, hence their name, "essential fatty acids." Most labels won't say if the total fat content is good or bad fat, so I would urge you to get your good fat intake from avocados, seeds, nuts, and fish.

BAD FAT FOOD is difficult to digest and can lead to weight gain. Saturated fat, which often is included on the nutrition breakdown, is known to raise levels of cholesterol and increase the risk of heart disease, so always watch out for that if it is listed.

SATURATED FATS are solid at room temperature (butter, lard) and found mainly in animal produce and dairy products, in hard and soft margarines, cooking fats, cakes, biscuits, savory snacks, and other processed foods, confectionaries, and chocolate.

TRANS FATS—the evil twin of saturated fats—are produced when vegetable and fish oils are hydrogenated to turn them into margarine or shortening. Like saturated fats from animal food, they block the conversion of essential fats, and research has shown that they may be even worse for you than saturated fats as they not only raise levels of bad blood cholesterol but also lower levels of good cholesterol. Low fat spreads often contain hydrogenated or partially hydrogenated fats.

Also be aware that LOW FAT FOODS often contain sugar to make up for the lack of flavor from the fats. If sugar is not used by the body for energy it can be converted into fat and stored just like fat, so there's no benefit in swapping to "low fat" if it simply means high sugar.

YOUR DIET PROFILE

Take your Food Diary and the packaging you have collected and create your own individual diet profile by following these simple steps. Evaluate the current reality and then write down how you'd like to improve each aspect of your diet, describing your goals.

1 PERCENTAGE OF FRESH FOOD VERSUS NON-FRESH

The first thing I want you to look at is the amount of fresh food you eat versus non-fresh. Is it about half and half, or more like 75 percent processed and 25 percent fresh? If you can eat a few more meals made from fresh ingredients, that would be a good change to make. Processed and refined foods are typically high in sugar, salt, saturated fat, trans fats, chemicals, additives, and preservatives, and low in nutrients. All these substances simply aren't good for you. By contrast, healthy fresh food is rich in the nutrients you need.

2 ARE YOU EATING YOUR FIVE PORTIONS OF VEGETABLES A DAY?

Vegetables are nutritional superstars. They are powerful sources of health- and immune-boosting antioxidants, vitamins, minerals, and phytochemicals that not only help you look and feel good, but also offer vital protection against all kinds of disorders and reduce the risk of diabetes, heart disease, and cancer. Vegetables also aid digestion and encourage the elimination of toxins and waste because of their fiber content. The question is, are you getting enough of them?

3 ARE YOU EATING THE SAME THINGS EVERY DAY?

When I see a Food Diary for the first time, one of the main things that strikes me is the lack of variety. Often people eat the same things every day, day in, day out. Even if you are eating a healthy food, you should not eat the same thing every single day. So if you like porridge oats, do not eat them seven mornings a week. It is easy to develop food sensitivities when you expose your body to the same food all the time. If you can, eat foods on a four-day rotation. So if you have porridge on a Monday, don't eat it again until Thursday.

4 ARE YOU JUNKING OUT?

How many fast-food orders, ready meals, or processed foods are you eating? Many are loaded with salt, sugar, colorings, additives, hardened (partially hydrogenated or hydrogenated) vegetable oil, and other hidden evils. Plus many of the good nutrients are processed out of these foods, so if you live on them you will literally be malnourished. Stop eating them. Junk foods are a direct assault on your body, increasing its toxic load and promoting obesity, heart disease, and other health problems.

5 ARE YOU A SUGAR JUNKIE?

Are you consuming sugar at breakfast, lunch, dinner, in your teas and coffees? Is it hidden in your cereal boxes, and are you adding more? Are you a soft drink fanatic? You must limit your intake of sugar, sweeteners, and sugary foods if you want to feel well and lose weight. Table sugar contains nothing more than empty calories and goes straight into your bloodstream. It causes rapid swings in blood sugar and energy levels. Natural sweeteners like fruit juice or fresh fruits are the best alternatives.

6 ARE YOU A SALT JUNKIE?

Too much salt in your diet may upset the sodium/potassium balance in your body and trigger high blood pressure and heart disease. Salty diets are also linked to fluid retention and kidney stones. The main sources of sodium in your diet are table salt, cooking salt, sauces, and processed foods. It's hidden in so many things. Steer clear of salty potato chips, and cured and smoked meats. Instead of adding salt to boost flavor, experiment with herbs and spices for alternatives. If you do use a very small amount of salt, then be sure to use sea salt.

7 DO YOU EAT ENOUGH RAW FRUITS AND VEGETABLES?

It is important to eat raw food every day. You will feel so much better if you increase your intake of raw foods. Are you eating raw foods as part of every meal? If not, then there's room for improvement! To include more raw in your diet:

► Make raw fruit smoothies in the mornings.
► Eat fruit salads.
► Snack on fruits.
► Include sprouted seeds like alfalfa sprouts in your salads.
► Every time you eat something cooked, always include some raw leaves, vegetables, or salad.
► In the colder months, when you may be eating more soups and stews, toss in lots of raw herbs and even raw veggies just before serving.
► In the warmer months, eat more raw foods. At least half your main meal should be raw.

8 IS THERE TOO MUCH WHEAT IN YOUR DIET?

Are you eating toast for breakfast every day, snacking on sandwiches, eating bread with dinner and toast for supper? Wheat contains gluten, which can lead to digestive problems in some and may interfere with metabolism in others. If you want to lose weight, you will have to go wheat-free for a while. And as part of a healthy, varied diet it's important to introduce other grains such as brown rice, barley, spelt, millet, amaranth, quinoa, and rye.

9 ARE YOU DRINKING ENOUGH WATER?

Your body is made up of two-thirds water, so water intake and distribution is vital for balancing hormones, eliminating waste products, keeping your cells working, and delivering nutrients to your organs. Dehydration is a sure way to help yourself put on weight. You need to drink at least six to eight glasses of water each day.

10 DO YOU EAT TOO MANY "WHITE" FOODS?

White pasta, white rice, and white bread are refined foods. They are not only low in nutrients but quick to release sugar. This means you may get a quick high followed by long slumps of energy. Cut them out.

11 COMPARE YOUR INTAKE OF GOOD FATS VERSUS BAD FATS

You should try to obtain as little fat as possible from saturated fats or trans fats found in animal products and processed foods and as much as possible in the form of essential fatty acids, particularly omega 3 and 6. Without sufficient quantities of EFAs your body cannot manufacture the hormones and chemicals you need to stay healthy, happy, and trim. So, in a nutshell, are you eating enough avocados, oily fish, olive oil, hemp oil, seeds, and nuts?

12 DO YOU USE HERBS AND SPICES?

Gentle spices and herbs add taste and variety to your food, and most have health benefits too. It's time to ditch the salt and pepper and be adventurous.

13 ARE YOU A CAFFEINE ADDICT?

Caffeine contains a chemical called benzoic acid which has a toxic and dehydrating effect on your body. Caffeine in tea, coffee, chocolate, and caffeinated soft drinks also acts as a stimulant and causes a fast rise in blood pressure and blood sugar, followed by a quick drop that contributes to a roller coaster ride of mood swings, fatigue, concentration problems, headaches, and anxiety. To top it all off, caffeine whips your adrenal glands into exhaustion, causing an imbalance in stress hormones. Poor adrenal function leaves you prone to putting on pounds around your middle, and it leaves you feeling wiped out. So, far from being a quick pick-me-up, caffeine just makes you feel tired, irritable, incontinent, and old before your time. Try caffeine-free herb teas instead.

14 ARE YOU EATING ORGANICALLY?

If you want to reduce the toxic load on your body, organic food is really the best way forward. The production of organic food is governed by strict standards and the use of chemicals and preservatives is avoided. Many supermarkets now sell organic food, but if you can't find or afford much organic food, remember that even if you eat organic food now and again or just stick to organic fruit and veggies it can still help to enhance your health.

15 HOW MUCH RED MEAT DO YOU EAT?

How often are you eating red meat? A diet heavy in high protein, fatty, red meat can be hard going on your digestion. It can deplete nutrients, overwork the kidneys and liver, cause digestive problems, and increase the proportion of harmful bacteria that live in your gut. Several studies link too much red meat to kidney stones, colon disorders, heart disease, and constipation. There is no red meat on my *Ultimate Health Plan* because I want to get your digestive system back in top working order. But this doesn't mean you can never eat red meat again. Personally, I don't eat meat, but if you want to make it an occasional food, that's fine. If you do, then make sure to buy organic, quality, lean, and trimmed meat and eat with lightly steamed green veggies and a salad of leaves and sprouted seeds.

16 WHERE ARE YOU EATING?

If you eat out a lot, are you choosing restaurants with good, healthy, quality foods? Are you making healthy choices when ordering? For example, opting for grilled fish instead of fried, or side vegetables instead of chips?

17 ARE YOU A NON-VEGGIE-EATING VEGETARIAN?

Removing meat from your diet and surviving on cheese sandwiches, potato chips, and beans on white toast is not going to hack it. I have met many vegetarians over the years who do not eat a balanced diet. They have stopped eating meat but seem to survive on lots of chips and junk foods. This is not a healthy way to live. If you want to be a vegetarian, you must learn how to do it properly. You need to eat widely from fruits, vegetables, seeds, nuts, beans, grains, legumes, seaweeds, sprouted seeds, sprouted nuts, and pulses, and possibly eggs and fish, depending on what kind of veggie you are. When properly planned, vegetarian diets are very healthy, and as a group, vegetarians are less likely to develop high blood pressure, diabetes, coronary heart disease, or obesity.

18 DO YOU EXERCISE MORE THAN THREE TIMES WEEKLY?

You need to move your butt every day. Exercise can boost energy in all kinds of ways. It increases circulation and by so doing helps lower LDL (bad) cholesterol and increase HDL (good) cholesterol.

Exercise:

► Can lower blood sugar levels and promote insulin efficiency—fatigue is a symptom of blood sugar imbalance.
► Keeps bowels working efficiently to eliminate waste products your body doesn't need or want and that can slow you down.
► Boosts immunity, which means you are less likely to get ill.
► Burns calories and builds up muscles. The more your muscles build up, the speedier your metabolism becomes.
► Encourages a good night's sleep.
► Improves your sex life.
► Boosts mood through the release of brain chemicals called endorphins.

19 ARE YOU SNACKING HEALTHILY AND REGULARLY?

Regular healthy snacking—for example fruit, nuts, seeds, or veggie sticks—is the key to keeping your blood sugar levels balanced. This means your energy levels stay high and your mood stays good. It also means that you don't ever feel hungry. If more than three or four hours is left between meals or snacks you're more likely to crave unhealthy, high-sugar foods because your blood sugar levels are low and your stomach is empty.

20 ARE YOU EATING ENOUGH FIBER A DAY?

Add fiber-rich foods to your diet like oats, fruit, seeds, vegetables, brown rice, and beans. Fiber is the bran of the grain, the cell walls of the vegetables, the pulp of the fruits. In other words it is the indigestible portion of these foods that improves intestinal function, helps to grow healthy bacteria in the gut, and helps to prevent disease by ensuring the removal of waste products and toxins. It also ensures that digestion is healthy and helps maintain blood sugar balance. Follow my Plan and you'll automatically get enough.

21 HOW MUCH OF YOUR DIET IS DAIRY?

Dairy products are high in saturated fat that can lead to weight gain and its associated problems if consumed in high quantities. I will take you off dairy on my Plan and even afterwards; if you want to have milk, try goat's milk, sheep's milk, or experiment with the vast array of grain milks such as rice and oat. Cow's milk is difficult for humans to digest, which is why so many people are lactose intolerant. Indigestibility can trigger an allergic response, bloating, diarrhea, flatulence, constipation, PMS, headaches, irritability, fatigue, and weight problems.

22 WHAT DO YOU EAT WHEN?

Missing breakfast and fasting most of the day, then eating a large dinner in the evening sends your body confusing signals. First of all, during the day when you are hardly eating, your body will slow down its metabolic rate to conserve energy. Then when you do eat in the evening your body is set up to store as much fat as possible. After eating, you often go to bed, so your body has little time to use up the calories you have just consumed. Eat during the day when you need the energy, not at night when activity levels are typically lower. In other words, are you focusing on eating a hearty breakfast and lunch and reducing your food intake at the end of the day? If you are eating a big dinner after 8:00 p.m., then expect to feel sluggish in the morning and to gain weight.

23 IS YOUR ENERGY LOW?

To access energy, it's crucial that your diet is rich in the nutrients your body needs to function optimally. Fatigue is often a symptom of blood sugar imbalances caused by poor eating habits, poor nutrient uptake, and nutrient deficiencies. And if you are eating rubbish a lot of the time, you increase your toxic load, which results in even more fatigue.

Energy Crash = Sugar Binges

When you feel low, a natural reaction is to reach for any kind of food to give you an energy boost. The problem is that, all too often, those foods are bad fat-laden, junky, sugary nonfoods that give you short-fuse energy zaps that are quickly followed by energy slumps and, eventually, weight gain.

24 ARE YOU STRESSING OUT?

Look through your Food Diary. Did you note any of the following?

- ▶ Salt or sugar cravings
- ▶ Feeling bloated after eating, or digestive problems
- ▶ Mid-afternoon energy slumps
- ▶ Constant hunger
- ▶ Emotional roller coaster rides, a short fuse, lack of concentration, crying, or feeling depressed, anxious, or impatient
- ▶ Insomnia or difficulty falling asleep
- ▶ Difficulty getting out of bed in the morning

Is stress making you fat? When you get stressed, your adrenal glands prompt the release of sugar stores into the bloodstream. If stress is prolonged, this sugar stays in your bloodstream, increasing the risk of blood sugar problems that can trigger weight gain. That's without eating anything sugary or fattening!

Think about how you live your life and what kinds of changes you could make to bring about balance. Is most of your life devoted to work-related activities? Are you exercising enough to sweat out your stress hormones? Getting some fun in your life is key to a healthy lifestyle.

25 ARE YOU DRINKING TOO MUCH ALCOHOL?

Alcohol stimulates your appetite and weakens your liver (your body's fat-burning powerhouse) and is full of sugar. The odd glass of wine here or there won't hurt, but if weight loss is your goal, forget about it until you reach your desired weight. It will be worth it.

Example Goals

- ► I want to be slim

- ► I want to banish my daily headaches

- ► I want to wake up with energy

- ► I want to sleep peacefully through the night

- ► I want brighter eyes

- ► I want radiant skin

- ► I want to feel more relaxed

- ► I want to be more energized in the afternoon

- ► I want to stop slumping in front of the TV every night

I want to stop eating junk
and start eating fresh, natural
foods full of goodness!

Look in the Mirror

The other morning, I delivered my children to school late because I needed to have a very long, drawn-out consultation to help the babysitter with something. As I was finally going out the door to go to work, my Mum called and said she absolutely had to talk to me that minute and it could not wait. Just as I managed to hang up, a friend called. She had just had a fight with her partner and needed a shoulder to cry on. I arrived at work late for a meeting, full of all the excuses of the day, blaming the babysitter, my mother, and my friend. I started to justify my tardiness, "If somebody calls me then how can I get to my next place on time?" A colleague observed that I needed boundaries and discipline and not excuses. Suddenly I realized I was blaming Mum, friend, and babysitter for my being Miss Tardy, and that just wasn't good enough.

When consulting with clients, the number of excuses for not eating properly is beyond a joke:

- My boyfriend likes pub grub.
- My girlfriend eats like a sparrow so there is nothing to eat in the fridge.
- My husband hates the taste of health food.
- My kids won't eat any of it.
- I don't have the time to do what you want, Gillian.
- It's all too expensive.

It is so easy to think of excuses. It's much harder to take responsibility for yourself.

- Stop blaming others for all the problems in your life.
- Stop blaming the fact that you have to go to work for having no time to prepare your food.
- Stop blaming your parents for your being overweight.
- Stop blaming your husband for influencing your salt intake with evening meals.
- Stop blaming the kids for your chocolate addiction.
- Just stop the Blame Game and start taking responsibility, now!

Visualizing Your Goals

Everything in life is about energy. Some types of energy are more obvious than others, for example electricity or radio waves. I am a great believer in the power of our own mental energy. Our thoughts and our written or spoken words and messages to ourselves are the keys to achieving our life dreams, and this invisible energy should not be underestimated.

Energy Goal Drawing

Now that you've mapped out your goals, by analyzing and
evaluating your own food and lifestyle habits and deciding what
you want to change, I want you to follow my Energy Goal Drawing
Exercise. I want to teach you how to harness energy and make your
goals happen. You are literally going to visualize success and
reach your potential.

1 START WITH A THOUGHT

What do you want? For instance, you may set an objective that you want to be slimmer, or have more energy or a radiant complexion.

EXAMPLE:

I WANT TO BE SLIMMER

2 WRITE DOWN YOUR THOUGHT

Once you commit your thought to paper, you elevate the thought to a new level of energy.

EXAMPLE:

I AM SLIM

3 ASSESS THE ACTION NEEDED TO ACHIEVE YOUR GOAL

Think about what it will take to become slim, healthy, or energized. Break it down into steps. For example, if your goal is to be slim, then your first Action Step is to keep a diary of everything you eat and drink for a week. Your second Action Step might be to throw away all the rubbish foods that I tell you are too nasty for your body. And so on.

EXAMPLE:

STEP 1. Create a Food Diary

STEP 2. Throw out all your rubbishy food

THIS IS ONLY AN EXAMPLE TO ILLUSTRATE THE POSSIBILITIES. I WANT YOU TO PLAN THIS OUT WITH YOUR INDIVIDUAL GOALS AND STEPS TO MATCH. BE CREATIVE AND DO ANYTHING HERE THAT MEETS YOUR OWN ASPIRATIONS.

4 DRAW YOUR GOAL IN A PICTURE

With a black pen, I want you to draw on plain, white paper whatever it is that you want to achieve or how you want to see yourself. So using the slim example, draw a simple figure of yourself looking slim and happy. You do not need to be Rembrandt. All you need to do is draw with stick figures. Put a caption underneath your drawing.

EXAMPLE:

(Your name) IS SLIM. I AM SLIM.

5 DRAW YOUR ACTION STEPS

With a black pen on white paper, draw pictures of you actually going through your Action Steps to reach your end goal.

EXAMPLE:

- A picture of a Food Diary with caption, "(Your name) fills out Food Diary."
- Complete the pictures and follow it through until you get to your end result and you are now slim.
- Our thoughts have powerful energy. When we write down these thoughts, and even transfer them into pictures, we dramatically intensify them. You are now harnessing the thought into action.
- You can make anything happen. You become the creator of your own destiny.
- Review your drawings every day and redraw them once a month.
- You may find that, on reflection, you wish to elaborate some steps or shorten some steps. After all, you now know that you are the creator of your own destiny.

PLEASE NOTE THAT THE EXAMPLES ABOVE ARE ALL IN THE PRESENT TENSE, WHICH FURTHER STRENGTHENS THE ENERGY OF YOUR THOUGHT. SO INSTEAD OF "I WILL BE SLIM" IT'S "I AM SLIM." THIS METHOD LEAVES NO ROOM FOR DOUBT. WHEN YOU STATE "I AM" THERE IS NOWHERE ELSE TO GO BUT GET RESULTS AND ACHIEVE SUCCESS.

EMBRACING CHANGE

After consulting with hundreds of clients over many years,
the greatest challenge I have faced as a nutritionist has been
to remove the barriers that most people erect for themselves.
We impede our own abilities to fly. We create blockages, doubts,
clouded perceptions, and negativity every day for ourselves that
need not be.

As a practitioner, this is a real problem for me. It can be
extremely difficult to tempt a closed soul to the magnificence
of new foods and a new lifestyle.

Are You Stagnant?

This is an issue about getting set in our ways, becoming stagnant, rigid, and blocked. Once we become set in our ways, we usually stay that way. If you have been eating fish and chips for the last 20 years, the chances are that you will feel most comfortable continuing on the same path. We usually choose the path of least resistance.

The goal in this section is to get your mind and body ready and open to accept change.

Emotional Blocks

Life is full of "stuff." Everyone goes through what I call life stuff, for example a relationship breakup, the child who disappoints, the mother who doesn't accept, the death of a loved one, an accident, illness, or stress. It is a part of the experience of life, but it also takes its toll on our energetic flow, whether we recognize it or not. By not recognizing it, we spur these blockages to new heights. Many people try all their lives to avoid facing their life stuff. "Don't want to talk about it. Just forget it. Life goes on."

Emotions and Your Body

It is this kind of emotional repression that causes disruption to the body's natural energetic meridians, possibly contributing to weight problems, digestive disorders, immune dysfunctions, constipation, backaches, irritable bowels, high blood pressure, migraines, diabetes, heart disease, indigestion, exhaustion, aches and pains, and worse. It is this same emotional holding and blockage that also causes us to become resistant to new ideas and so frightened of accepting new foods, however delicious or healthy.

Getting Back to Basics

By simply taking note of your blocked energy, you help to dissolve it. When we recognize and acknowledge disturbed energy, instead of hiding from, ignoring, or running away from it, we are able to process it through our systems and let it go.

Using the following exercises, I have been able to get clients to (a) become more open in thought and accepting of new foods and new lifestyles; (b) jump-start the eradication of some fundamental health complaints; and (c) spark a healing, revitalization, and wellness process.

It may all sound a bit far-fetched but all I require is that you do the exercises and then see for yourself the changes that could take place.

Peel an Onion

I want you to get an onion and start to peel away the layers. Keep peeling away the layers until you get to the core, the center. We all have a core essence. In the children's animated film *Shrek*, the big, green, crusty ogre laments that he will never get to his original self. He is disillusioned, dissatisfied, jaded, disappointed, frustrated, skeptical, and angry at the world. He is so overloaded with layers of onion that his original core can never be resurrected, he worries. But once Shrek begins to love himself, he discovers that his true self is really kind, cuddly, cool, and beautiful.

So, when you peel the onion, it represents the layers of buildup that you may have held on to as you've gone through life. The way in which you reacted to various experiences, whatever they may have been, perhaps crusted you over and left you more resistant and less open to change. You can peel back the layers and find your original self. Keep reminding yourself of what the onion peeling represents. Feel yourself becoming more open and willing to accept change and new concepts. Recognize the layers but then move on.

Opening Up Emotionally for Change

So you have peeled the onion. Now I want you to access your center and open up your body for change. Many new medical and scientific studies now prove that our body's cells and molecules listen to the messages that we express and respond accordingly. If we constantly tell ourselves negative statements like we are "too tired," "too old," "too ill," "too fat," "over the hill," "past our prime," or that we "can't lose the weight," "can't get the job," "can't find love," and so on, our body will listen and ultimately adopt the same attitude in a downward spiral.

Being able to open up emotionally in order to accept change, especially when it comes to the food habits of a lifetime, is about learning how to create your own new messages. Talking nicely to yourself really works. When the body is in harmony with itself and its environment, our energies work like a charm to help promote a healthy system. And so for starters, I never allow my clients to use the word "can't," so neither can you.

We only CAN DO!

EMBRACE YOUR NEW LIFESTYLE

A plethora of new research now definitively confirms that emotions and physiology are intricately linked and strongly dependent upon each other. We cannot ignore one or the other: the physical and the emotional are both essential to a healthy lifestyle.

In order to be more receptive and cultivate an attitude of openness toward a change of lifestyle, thereby accepting an abundance of new foods, do the following exercise once or twice daily, first thing in the morning and again in the evening:

1. Sit squarely on a firm chair with feet planted on the floor; feel your feet touching the ground.

2. Count up from 1 to 10, closing your eyes, and just relax.

3. With eyes closed, listen to the gentle sound of your breath.

4. Breathe through your nose. As you slowly inhale, imagine that you are filling your whole body internally with oxygen, from your toes to the top of your head.

5. Exhale slowly. Repeat for a couple of minutes, imagining the oxygen flowing through all the cells of your body.

6. Then bring both hands up to your chest, and hold your palms flat against your chest. Feel your palms on your chest as you breathe. Sit like this for a couple of minutes.

7. You may then place your hands by your side, and say the following, silently to yourself or softly aloud, three times very slowly:

"I open myself to enjoy a whole new array of foods."

8. Once you have finished saying the above sentence to yourself, then begin to count down from 10 to 1 and slowly open your eyes.

THE EXCUSE PROMISE

Get a notepad and make a list of the reasons you have used in the past to stop you from improving your health, eating habits, and lifestyle choices. Identify routines, habits, or lifestyle choices that you have used as a reason for not making positive changes in your life. Here are some of the excuses I have heard over the years:

- **Stressful lifestyle**
- **Too busy**
- **Partner has unhealthy eating habits**
- **Family too demanding, so no energy for myself**
- **Don't know where to start**
- **Too expensive**

Once you have acknowledged your excuses, write the following sentences on your notepad:

I no longer allow any of the above excuses to stop me from achieving my potential. I am free to do anything if I set my mind to it.

Know that the healthier you keep your body and mind, the easier it will be to cope with a demanding lifestyle. Regardless of how unhealthily a partner eats, you do not have to follow that person's bad habits. If your partner encourages you to eat unhealthily, you need to explain to him or her that you are concerned about your health and need to make changes. But you can never blame anyone else for your situation. You cannot blame your hubby for your chocolate cravings or your junk food habits. If your partner doesn't want to go along with you, then you do it for yourself. Let them do whatever they do. But do not let anyone hold you back from changing your life for the better. Positive change can fit into any lifestyle, no matter how busy. Identifying your excuses is an important start.

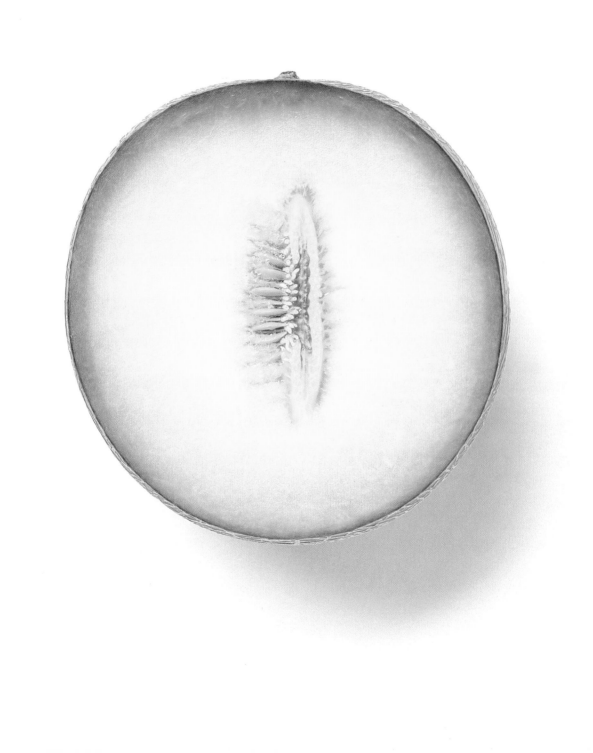

BREAKING BAD HABITS

A habit is something you do repeatedly, over and over. There is
no set number of times you need to do something for it to become
a habit. It becomes a habit when you do it automatically (without
really thinking), and when challenged about the habit, you find
it difficult to change. You may even become defensive.

You Are What You Choose to Be

Choice gives you the ability to break bad habits. You always have
a choice. You can be a lousy eater and feel dreadful as a result of
your poor food choices, or you can choose to eat the right foods and
realize your health potential.

Magic Bullets

You can create your own magic bullet for change by following
the steps outlined on the following pages.

STEP 1 IDENTIFY YOUR BAD HABITS

To break bad habits, you need to first of all become aware of what they are. This brings them back into the realm of consciousness and helps you regain your ability to make choices.

Grab a pen and paper and write a list of all the things you do that you know are not good for you, even if you enjoy doing them. For example, eating foods high in sugar and fat, indulging in ice cream, not getting enough exercise, smoking, and so on.

STEP 2 WHAT'S IN IT FOR YOU?

What's the motivation for doing something that is bad for you? Why do you do it? Ask yourself why you find this action so compelling. In other words, what's your payoff for doing something that you know isn't good for you? There is always a payoff. But is the payoff worth it? For example, let's say your bad habit is to snack on several bars of chocolate a day. Okay, you get a quick comfort fix when you eat it. But how long does that last? Instead of doing any exercise, you get to slob out in front of the TV. The payoff is probably that you get to unwind and relax. But there are other ways of doing that too.

STEP 3 ARE YOU TRADING OFF?

Analyze the trade-off. What is it that you are losing by giving in to your habit? This step should be easier. Why is it that you consider it a bad habit in the first place? Eating too much chocolate is a bad habit because it interferes with your blood sugars and triggers mood swings, and it also encourages weight gain. Not exercising enough is a bad habit because it makes you feel unfit and out of shape. In both cases you are trading short-term comfort for long-term weight gain and poor health and well-being. When you look at it that way, it doesn't seem like you are making very wise choices, does it? There has to be a better way.

STEP 4 PAYOFF OR TRADE-OFF—THAT IS THE QUESTION

Now that you've looked at both sides of the issue—your payoff and your trade-off, indulging in a bad habit is no longer an involuntary act. You now know that you are making a choice every time you perform this action. So each time you feel tempted to indulge in a bad habit, remind yourself that you have a choice here. Which do you value more? Do you value more the instant relief you get from snacking unhealthily or slobbing in front of the TV, or do you value your overall health and well-being more? I want you to become more conscious and aware. Don't go through life unengaged with yourself, mindlessly going through the motions and stuffing rubbish into yourself. If you make conscious choices then you will most likely make the right choices.

If you listen to your body and make intuitive food choices then you will make the right choices.

STEP 5 SUBSTITUTING BETTER HABITS

The reason you formed your habits in the first place is that they may have filled a need. Some people say that they needed to feel comforted, so they reached for bad food. Maybe you were feeling tired, so you switched the TV on for the whole evening. I want you to start making active choices to break these old patterns and not fall into the old action. You will be making a choice to perform a better, alternative action in its place. Instead of grabbing a chocolate bar when you feel low, eat an apple or decide to call a friend; write a letter or have a warm bath when you feel tense. Instead of switching the TV on the minute you come in at night, go for a walk. Which new habit you adopt is not so relevant. What's important is whether you feel good about the choices you have made. After all, the reason you consider it a bad habit is because it leaves you feeling bad about yourself.

STEP 6 IT'S UP TO YOU

The only way to give bad habits a lifeline is to sink back into denial about why you have bad habits in the first place. Each time you begin to resume your old patterns, the thought will pass through your mind that you are trading one thing for another each time you perform that action. You will be forced to make a choice about continuing your habit. What choices will you make? The one that makes you feel disappointed with yourself or the one that makes you feel positive about yourself? It's up to you. To empower yourself, make the choice that you know intuitively is the right one.

DUMP THE JUNK

This is the scary part when you get to invite Dr. Gillian McKeith into your home. We need to get to the bottom of what's really lurking in your cupboards, have a good clear out, and then start afresh.

You have already kept and analyzed your Food Diary for seven days, plus inventoried a week's worth of packaging from all that you have eaten.

So now that you know what you need to dump, let's get to it! Just in case there is any confusion, here's a checklist of what to clear out for the duration of the Plan:

- **Alcohol (does it help if I tell you that alcohol causes cellulite?)**
- **Butter**
- **Caffeinated drinks (coffee, black tea, colas)**
- **Cakes and biscuits**
- **Canned foods with added sugar and salt**
- **Carbonated drinks**
- **Chocolates or chocolate bars**
- **Cow's milk**
- **Cream**
- **Hard cheeses**
- **Hot spicy foods (such as chili sauces)**
- **Ice cream**
- **Margarine and lard**
- **Packaged foods with added sugar or salt**
- **Pastries**
- **Pizzas**
- **Potato chips**
- **Processed meats (including bacon, ham, and sausages)**
- **Ready meals**
- **Red meat**
- **Refined white sugar**
- **Sweets**
- **Table salt**
- **Wheat products**
- **White bread products**
- **White pasta**
- **White rice**

Now I know what you are thinking: *There is nothing left to eat!* Don't be depressed about this list, it looks worse than it really is.

It is a wrench at first, but it's just fantastic that you are making this change. You are going to eat more foods than you thought imaginable. There will be so many new choices that you will be dazzled to the core. It really is a celebration of food that is going to turn your life around.

It's also worth knowing now that once you make these changes for a sustained period of time, your body will start to adjust. In effect, you may even become repelled by the bad food and actually crave only good foods. Okay, on the surface, you may think this is a mad Gillian mirage, but I must tell you it is attainable.

I do not expect you to dump the entire list forever in eternity. I only demand full compliance for the duration of my Plan, no questions asked! I'm hoping you'll even enjoy it—just think of the fresh start.

level two
the ultimate health plan

You are now in the thick of it and ready to embark on my 28-day plan. The good news is that if you need to lose weight then you will with my new lifestyle. Everyone knows the results I get. And for even better results, do my two-day Fat Flush or Detox (Level Three) first. If you simply want to feel more healthy then my Ultimate Health Plan will work just as brilliantly for you too. Whether you want to lose weight or not, YOU ARE NOT ON A DIET. You have to throw away all previous ideas about diets. With my program you are going to eat more foods than ever before without guilt or denial. And to get started, all you have to do is follow the Plan day by day. You do what I tell you and you succeed. It's that simple. But if you don't, then you lose the game.

   You will have to do it my way to the letter of my law. To repeat: it's my way or the highway. Easy.

COMPREHENSIVE FOOD LIST

When I look at the first-time Food Diaries of new clients who come to me wanting to lose weight, one thing strikes me every single time. They eat more or less the same 10 to 12 foods day in, day out, week in, week out, month in, month out. "Don't you ever get sick of eating the same foods every single day?" I query. The standard answer is that they don't realize they are eating the same old foods. Bad ones at that.

So, my goal for you is that you tantalize your palate and experience more good, healthy foods than you ever thought possible. Just when you thought there was nothing left to eat, feast your eyes on my list of the best foods to include in your life.

FISH

Carp
Cod
Dover sole
Flounder
Haddock
Hake
Halibut
Herrings
John Dory
Lemon sole
Mackerel
Monkfish
Orange roughy
Pollack
Red mullet
Salmon
Sardines
Sea bass
Sea bream
Snapper
Trout
Whitefish

LEAFY GREEN VEGETABLES

Arugula
Beet greens
Chard
Cress
Dandelion flowers
Dandelion greens
Endive
Escarole
Iceberg lettuce
Kale
Lamb's lettuce
Little gem lettuce
Loose-leaf lettuce
Mustard greens
Parsley, flat and
  curly
Romaine
Sorrell
Spinach
Swiss chard
Turnip greens
Watercress

VEGETABLES

Acorn squash
Artichoke
Asparagus
Avocado
Beets
Bok choy
Broccoli
Brussels sprouts
Butternut squash
Carrots
Cassava
Cauliflower
Celeriac
Celery
Chinese cabbage
Cucumber
Daikon
Eggplant
Fennel
Globe artichoke
Green cabbage
Green peas
Horseradish
Jerusalem artichoke
Kobocha squash
Kohlrabi
Leeks
Okra
Olives

Onions
Parsnips
Peppers
Purple sprouting
  broccoli
Radish
Red cabbage
Rutabaga
Salsify
Sauerkraut
Savoy cabbage
Scallions
Shallots
Shitake mushrooms
Snow peas
Squash
Sugar snap peas
Sweetcorn
Sweet potatoes
Tomatoes: yellow,
  orange, and red
Turnip
Uchiki kuri
White cabbage
Yams
Zucchini

SPROUTS

Beansprouts
Sprouted alfalfa
Sprouted chickpeas
Sprouted clover
Sprouted mung
   beans
Sprouted quinoa
Sprouted sunflower
   seeds
Any sprouted seed
   or nut

BEANS

Adzuki beans
Black beans
Borlotti beans
Butter beans
Cannellini beans
Carob chickpeas
Edamame (steamed
   soybeans)
Fava beans
Flageolet beans
Garbanzo beans
Great Northern
   beans
Green beans
Lentils, brown and
   red
Lima beans
Mung beans
Navy beans
Pinto beans
Soybeans
String beans

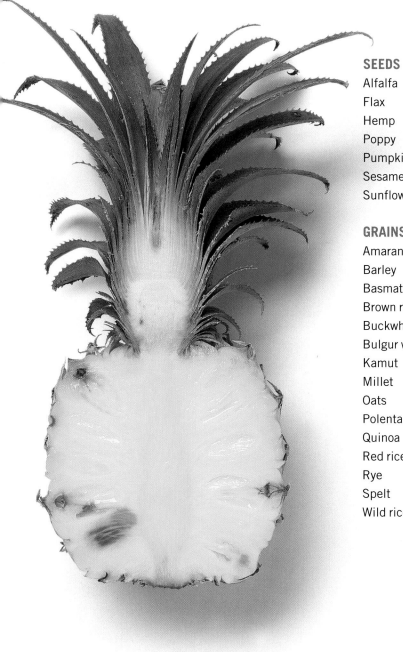

SEEDS
Alfalfa
Flax
Hemp
Poppy
Pumpkin
Sesame
Sunflower

GRAINS
Amaranth
Barley
Basmati rice
Brown rice
Buckwheat
Bulgur wheat
Kamut
Millet
Oats
Polenta
Quinoa
Red rice
Rye
Spelt
Wild rice

FLOURS
Amaranth flour
Buckwheat flour
Chickpea flour
Gram flour
Lentil flour
Oat flour
Potato flour
Rice flour
Rye flour
Soy flour
Spelt flour
Sunflower seed flour
Tapioca flour
Yellow corn flour

SEA VEGETABLES (SEAWEEDS)
Arame
Dulse
Hijiki
Kelp
Kombu
Nori sea lettuce
Sea palm
Wakame

CONDIMENTS

Brown rice vinegar
Cider vinegar
Miso paste
Miso powder
Mustard
Red wine vinegar
Sauerkraut
Tamari
Umeboshi plum
   sauce
Umeboshi vinegar
White wine vinegar

FRESH HERBS +
SPICES (FOR SEASONING)

Agar
All Spice
Aniseed
Basil
Bay leaves
Cardamom
Cayenne
Celery seeds
Chervil
Chives
Cinnamon
Cloves
Coriander
Cumin
Dill
Fenugreek
Garlic
Ginger
Mace
Marjoram
Mint
Mustard seeds
Nutmeg
Oregano
Parsley
Pepper
Rosemary
Saffron
Sage
Star Anise
Tarragon
Thyme
Turmeric
Vanilla pods

RAW NUTS

Almonds
Brazil nuts
Cashews
Chestnuts
Filberts
Hazelnuts
Pecans
Pine nuts
Pistachios
Walnuts

FRUIT

Apples
Apricots
Avocados
Bananas
Blackberries
Black currants
Blueberries
Cherries
Coconut
Cranberries
Currants
Damsons
Dates
Dried fruits
Elderberries
Figs
Gooseberries
Grapefruit, pink and
   white
Grapes
Greengages
Guavas
Kiwis
Kumquats
Lemons
Limes
Loganberries
Loquats
Lychees
Mandarins
Mangoes
Mulberries
Nashi pears
Nectarines
Papayas
Passion fruit
Papaws
Peaches
Pears
Persimmons
Pineapples
Plantains
Plums
Pomegranates
Prickly pears (cactus
   fruit)
Prunes
Quince
Raspberries
Red currants
Rhubarb
Sharon fruit
Star fruit
Strawberries
Tamarind
Tangerines
Ugli fruit

Melons

Banana melon
Cantaloupe
Galia
Honeydew
Watermelon

SWEETENERS

Agave syrup
Almond extract
Barley malt extract
Brown rice syrup
Carob amazake
Malt extract
Maple syrup
Mirin
Molasses
Vanilla extract

HERBAL TEAS

Borage
Chamomile
Dandelion
Fennel
Ginger
Ginseng
Hawthorn
Horsetail
Lemon balm
Liquorice
Melissa
Nettle
Pau d'arco

Peppermint
Red clover
Red raspberry
Rose hip
Slippery elm
Spearmint
Valerian root

Chicken
Turkey
Tofu
Tempeh
Soy
Yogurt

DR. GILLIAN'S FAVORITE WEIGHT LOSS FOODS

Adzuki beans
Apples
Avocados
Beet greens
Blueberries
Brown rice
Cardamom
Cucumbers
Dandelion greens
Dandelion tea
Flaxseed
Fruit smoothies

Ginger
Grapes
Leafy greens
Miso soup
Nettle tea
Oats
Oily fish
Papayas
Parsley
Pears
Pink grapefruit
Plums

Quinoa
Raw shelled hemp seeds
Raspberries
Seaweeds: nori, kombu,
    wakame, dulse
Soaked almonds
Sprouted seeds: chickpeas,
    alfalfa, sunflower seeds,
    mung beans, clover
Vegetable juices
Water

Dr. Gillian's Food Combo Rules

1. Fruit first, never for dessert.
2. Separate dense proteins from dense carbs at the same meal;
no chicken and rice together or fish and potatoes together.

Dr. Gillian's Top 20 Weight Loss Tips

1 EAT MORE, NOT LESS

Eating less than is required to support your basal metabolism will slow your metabolism down. My clients raise their metabolism and keep blood sugar levels stable with regular healthy eating. It also helps to prevent bingeing because you never feel famished.

2 SNACKING IS GOOD!

Watch out for the late afternoon and evening slump. If you want to burn fat and prevent your body from putting it back on, you must stabilize your blood sugar. In order to do this, you need to eat every two to three hours, which includes healthy snacking mid-morning and mid-afternoon. Fasting, skipping meals, or overly restrictive diets will enable you to lose weight but only in the short term. The weight you primarily lose is water weight and muscle tissue. When you restrict your food intake, your body instinctively thinks it's being starved and shifts into a protective mode by slowing down your metabolism and storing nearly all your calories as body fat. Losing muscle is the last thing you want.

3 DRINK MORE ... WATER

Drink eight glasses of water a day between meals. Have
a large glass of water 20 to 30 minutes before meals. Other
drinks to include are herbal teas and vegetable juices. If you
are exercising you should be drinking even more. Soft drinks,
juices, and teas and coffees full of caffeine don't count. Lack
of water can slow the metabolic rate just as lack of food can.
Since water is the body's most important nutrient, the liver
will turn its attention to water retention instead of doing
other duties such as burning fat. Dehydration, because
it causes headaches, lack of concentration, and fatigue,
is also often mistaken for hunger.

4 DON'T DRINK TOO MUCH WITH YOUR MEALS

Do not drink copious amounts of liquids with meals, not
even still water. Have a glass of water about half an hour
before you eat and take only little sips during meals if
you must. Soft drinks are banned.

5 EAT SOUP FIRST

Have soup before a meal. Studies show that soup before
a meal is a good way to feel satisfied.

6 FIND OUT WHAT'S EATING YOU

Eating foods that aren't healthy can often be triggered
by stress, boredom, loneliness, anger, depression, and other
emotions. Learning to deal with emotions without food
is a significant skill that will greatly serve long-term
weight control.

7 SLOW DOWN

Eating slowly is one method that can help take off pounds.
That's because from the time you begin eating, it takes the
brain 20 minutes to start signaling feelings of fullness. Fast
eaters often eat beyond their true level of fullness before the
20-minute signal has had a chance to set in. So slow down,
take smaller bites, and savor every tasty morsel. Nutrient
uptake is more effective too. When you wolf down your food, you
are not able to digest your food nutrients as effectively. Eating
too quickly can overload your stomach, causing gas and
bloating. Also you tend to gulp more air when you eat quickly.
So remember to eat regular meals and eat them slowly to
release the food nutrients properly.

8 EAT AT THE TABLE

Sit at the table when it's time to eat. I want you to focus
on what you are eating, and sitting on the sofa in front of the
TV is about as mindless as it gets. At the table, you will
eat more slowly and feel more full; and sitting up straight helps
digestion. Don't be a mindless muncher!

9 KEEP MOVING

Walking to the shops, mowing the lawn, and taking the stairs at work all count and keep you moving throughout the day. See pages 74–84 for my exercise program and also remember that the more you move, the more pounds you will lose.

10 DON'T SHOP WHEN YOU'RE HUNGRY

You'll end up buying all kinds of foods you know you shouldn't eat. Eat something before you go, make a shopping list, and stick to it.

11 BE PREPARED

Be prepared in order to avoid temptation. Take healthy lunches and snacks to work such as fruit, vegetable sticks and dips, soups, salads, bean sprouts, nuts, seeds, rye bread, oat cakes, avocados, peanut butter, leftovers from dinner, and herbal tea bags.

12 EAT IN THE RAW

Every time you have something cooked, eat something raw with it. Even if you make soup, you must add raw herbs or vegetables at the end. Raw foods are the only source of food enzymes, a catalyst for weight balance.

13 BLEND THE DAY AWAY

Eat lots of blended soups, such as sweet potato and squash. These are easy to digest. Fruit smoothies are great too. Make them for breakfast.

Weight Loss Helper Guide:

VITAMIN B COMPLEX Essential for efficient metabolism of carbs and proteins. Take 50mg daily.

ASTRAGALUS Packed with Vitamin B, it enhances adrenal function that is critical for weight loss. Get it in tincture form, put into hot water, and drink. Take 15 drops twice daily for three months.

SIBERIAN GINSENG Helps to stabilize blood sugar and diminish cravings. Take 15 drops twice daily for three months.

CO-ENZYME Q10 Helps stimulate the metabolism and weight loss. Take 150mg daily.

DIGESTIVE ENZYME SUPPLEMENTS Help boost nutrient uptake and suppress appetite. One with lunch and one with dinner.

RAW SHELLED HEMP SEEDS AND OIL Provides exactly the right combination of essential fatty acids to boost metabolism and weight loss. Take 1 or 2 tablespoons of seeds daily or every other day. Drizzle 1 tablespoon of oil over a raw salad.

KELP Helps support the thyroid gland and aid weight loss. Follow directions on the label.

ALOE VERA JUICE Has a soothing effect on the stomach. Take before meals and follow instructions on the label.

DR. GILLIAN McKEITH'S LIVING FOOD ENERGY POWDER Packed full of vitamins, enzymes, minerals, antioxidants, amino acids, essential fatty acids, and cofactors. Add 1 or 2 teaspoons a day to water or fruit juice.

LECITHIN GRANULES Helps utilize body fat. You can sprinkle them over salads. Take 2 teaspoons once a week.

CHICKWEED Helps break down fat deposits that are hard to shift. Take 15–30 drops of the tincture or 500mg capsule daily (before meals).

NETTLE TEA A great weight loss tea as it boosts metabolism and is a natural appetite suppressant. Alternate with dandelion tea and drink 3–4 cups daily.

RED RASPBERRY LEAF TEA May help to reduce appetite and tastes good.

SPIRULINA Rich in protein, this can help control blood sugar swings and food cravings. Take 6 tablets daily or 1 teaspoon of the powder form mixed in juice.

NOTE: ALWAYS CONSULT WITH YOUR GP BEFORE TAKING SUPPLEMENTS.

15 BREAKFAST LIKE A KING

Eat breakfast like a king, lunch like a queen, and dinner like a pauper. Make sure you eat more at lunchtime than for dinner.

16 EARLY TO BED

Get to bed by 10:30 p.m. Your liver and gallbladder need to do their detoxing work between 11:00 p.m. and 2:00 a.m. Healthy livers help balance weight. Studies show that sleeping before midnight and having regular sleeping and waking times is healthiest for the body. You need a good eight hours of sleep. Being tired slows your metabolism and can affect your food choices, making you go for high-calorie, fatty foods for a fast, brief energy burst.

17 EAT AT REGULAR TIMES

Try to eat breakfast, lunch, dinner, and snacks around the same time each day. Irregular eating habits can cause bloating. If you leave your stomach empty for long periods of time the secretion of digestive enzymes slows down. Irregular eating habits can also play havoc with your blood sugar, and you need a stable blood sugar level to keep you from gaining weight.

18 EAT DINNER EARLY

Dinner should be no later than 6:00 to 7:00 p.m., if possible. Unless you want to gain weight and feel sluggish, of course.

19 EAT WHEN CALM

If you are upset, wait until the feeling passes or lessens and then eat. Do not attempt to eat a full meal if you are stressed out or upset. Best to opt for vegetable juices or simple soups that day as they are much easier on the digestion.

20 THROW OUT YOUR SCALES

In all the years that I have been working with people who want to lose weight, I have never weighed anybody. People are too obsessed with weight. I don't do the weight thing, nor do I encourage calorie counting or portion controlling. Instead, I put you on a whole new lifestyle. You don't need to be a biophysicist or a mathematician to embark upon my journey.

If you want to have a positive, passionate relationship with food, you have to look at food in a whole different way. My Plan will allow your body to find its natural weight. But depriving yourself and saving up calories for unhealthy foods is a recipe for disaster. Give up the weighing and counting and release yourself.

THE SMOOTHIE SEMINAR

I consider myself the Queen of Smoothies. It's my number one choice for breakfast. My best friends make fun of me because my blender works overtime. If you come into my kitchen, you hear constant whirring as I blend and blend. In meetings, I often have a smoothie, on trains I always have containers of smoothies. I absolutely love to make them because they are so easy to toss together, they fill you up, are a cinch to digest, and taste delicious.

Smoothies are the perfect introduction to healthy eating. Low-cal, low fat, and high energy, they make a wonderful breakfast, light meal, or snack. So to give yourself a really easy way in to the Dr. Gillian lifestyle, think smoothies and get your blenders to the ready!

Good smoothies are generally thick and full-bodied. I like mine to have a pudding consistency, almost like yogurt. Juicers extract only the juice from fruit and leave the pulp behind—with a smoothie you use a blender and nothing goes to waste. They are so easy to prepare and so good for you. For example, throw into a blender a ripe peach or nectarine, a banana, and some strawberries, then blend for a minute or so, and voilà! You've got the hang of it. You are done!

Just be creative. The key is to experiment and have fun with it. And if you prefer to make your smoothie thinner, just add extra water or a watery fruit. You could even try adding a grain milk for an all-natural super smoothie milkshake. Or add a sprinkle of cinnamon for extra taste. Whatever you fancy.

EXERCISE

Have you ever noticed that when you are greeted by someone their first sentence is often, "Take a seat?" Why are we so obsessed with sitting? Every single person I have ever met who wants to lose weight does not move nearly enough. They get inside their cars and sit. They go to work and sit at a desk, then they go home and sit again. Our bodies are not designed to sit on sofas, slump at desks, slob out in front of the television, or stare at a computer screen hour after hour without moving. We need to transform ourselves from a nation of sitters to a nation of movers and shakers. The acceptance of a sedentary life is downright wrong, and we must change it.

Exercise is something that needs to be done continuously, all the time, every day. It's not enough to just fit it in once or twice a week, although even that's preferable to no exercise at all. I want you to move your body as much as you possibly can, throughout the day. This part of my lifestyle is non-negotiable. I am not asking you to become a fitness fanatic, but if you want to be slim and healthy then you need a positive attitude to exercise. I won't hear any excuses. There is no getting around me on this!

Break the Vicious Cycle

Lack of exercise is one of the most serious health issues facing the Western world today. And lack of movement is a vicious cycle. The less you move, the less you want to move and the less you are ultimately able to move.

When you eat the new Dr. Gillian way, you are introducing many more nutrients, vitamins, minerals, amino acids, proteins, phytonutrients, and essential fatty acids into your body and cells. The only truly effective way to properly distribute all of these new nutrients throughout your system is via exercise. Exercising before meals increases metabolism and enables you to burn your food more effectively. Once you start this good habit, you will not want to stop it.

Your new lifestyle should include a consistent attitude toward exercise—you should always be looking to keep active: cycle to the shops, walk to the supermarket, take the stairs, jog to the cinema, dance to music every night, stretch and skip rope outside, buy a hula hoop and learn to use it, or bounce on a trampoline.

On the Plan you need to incorporate some form of exercise into your everyday life. I'm not expecting you to be a fitness fanatic, but even 30 minutes a day of moderate activity will reap huge rewards. Regular exercise:

▶ **Gets your circulation going and makes you feel alive**
▶ **Speeds up metabolism and helps burn fat**
▶ **Releases endorphins that improve mood**
▶ **Increases your energy levels and improves sleep patterns**
▶ **Improves overall fitness and your ability to fight off colds and minor ailments**
▶ **Makes you feel good about yourself**

YOUR EXERCISE COMMITMENT

I require three exercise commitments from you. Place your signature in the box provided under each statement. This is your promise to me and to yourself.

One:
I agree to move my body every day through exercise.
Signature ....

Some days you may move and exercise more than other days. The important thing is that you do move.

Two:
I agree to exercise before each meal.

Signature ....

This can be as simple as brisk walking. You walk for 20 minutes before breakfast, 20 minutes before lunch, and walk or dance for 20 minutes before dinner. Or you might run in place or jump up and down on a mini trampoline for 10 minutes before your meal. (You may need to work up gradually to a full 20-minute walk or 10-minute run or trampoline.)

Three:
I agree to use a mini trampoline, swim, or join and use a gym regularly.

Signature ....

This is your insurance policy against bad weather. I don't want to hear that it was raining and you could not walk anywhere. If you are seriously overweight, you may have to lose a certain amount before you can get on a mini trampoline. In the meantime, try swimming. The water supports your body and takes all the stress off your joints while you concentrate on working those muscles. Joining a gym can be a fantastic motivator and a good way to meet like-minded people. Of course, you have to actually go to the gym and use it. Maybe two or three days a week you go to the gym, and you do some other exercise on the other days.

PLEASE NOTE:

Common sense is key here. If you are over 50, have any medical conditions, are pregnant, are very overweight, or have not exercised regularly for a long time, go and talk to your doctor about what sort of exercise regimen would be right for you. Listen to your body, and adjust your regimen to how you feel physically. Obviously, if you are unwell then you may need to lay off exercise. Or if your newborn baby was crying into the wee hours of the night and keeping you awake, then you may wish to reduce your fitness plan for the next morning. Gauge it for yourself and talk to your doctor. There may be days here and there where you do a little less or you do more.

Do It Daily

You need to do something every day, no matter how small. Depending on your starting weight and stamina, do 1 minute, work up to 5 minutes, 10 minutes, then 15 minutes. Gradually and slowly work up to at least 30 minutes and then up to an hour, four to six times a week. But you should still move on the seventh day. Some days you can do more or less exercise than others. So maybe five days a week you are doing some form of exercise for up to an hour a day, and on the other two days you are doing only 20 minutes. Are you catching my point here? I want you to adapt the exercise to your abilities and also how you are feeling on that particular day. Our bodies are very dynamic organisms, and we need to adjust to that dynamism. The old adage, "No pain, no gain," does not apply here. My exercise program is not about hurting or killing your body. I want your exercise to be in harmony and in tune with your muscles, endurance levels, and frame.

Often, when they hear me give a seminar, people get excited about an exercise program. After 20 years of not moving, they want to jog for miles right away. This could be a great way to do yourself in. This type of person might be incapacitated for weeks because they have weakened their body and stressed their muscles. The aches and pains will be harrowing. This is not what I want.

Stick with It

Getting to 30 minutes of exercise and eventually up to an hour or more five, six, or seven times a week may take several weeks or even a few months to achieve. Just stick with it and you'll soon find that your fitness levels and your enjoyment will increase. If you don't think you can find a spare 30 minutes or so at one time, try to include several short bouts of activity in a day, say three 10-minute sessions at first, working up to three 20-minute sessions. You are then exercising for an hour a day. Exercise must be:

▶ **Consistent**
▶ **Performed every single day in some form**
▶ **Varied**
▶ **Adapted to how you feel that day**

WHAT KIND OF EXERCISE?

A combination of aerobic exercise and resistance/flexibility training is ideal:

▶ **Aerobic—walking, jogging, swimming, cycling, rowing, dancing, skating, trampolining**
▶ **Resistance and flexibility—yoga, Pilates, weights, resistance exercises (such as press ups)**

My best advice is to vary the exercise for two reasons:

1. It is better for the muscles and the body.
2. It prevents boredom and keeps you more interested.

EXERCISE PLAN FOR BEGINNERS

Walking

Walking is one of my favorite forms of exercise. No expertise or equipment is required. You can do it anytime and it's free! Provided you do it regularly and for long enough, walking can be just as beneficial as any of the more vigorous activities (like jogging or trampolining).

HOW TO START

Take a 10-minute walk, twice a day. Gradually extend yourself:

► Walk every day
► Walk longer
► Walk faster
► Walk and swing your arms at the same time
► Walk up one or two gentle slopes
► Walk up steeper slopes

Ideally I would like you to work up to walking for one hour. You can break that hour up into three sets of 20 minutes: 20 minutes before breakfast, 20 minutes before lunch, and 20 minutes before dinner.

Swimming

For most people, especially those who are very overweight, swimming is even better than walking. Start by going to the pool twice a week for a gentle 15-minute swim. When I swim, I count the number of laps I swim. Start with one lap of the pool and comfortably and gradually increase the number of laps and your work rate while in the water. Aim to build up to about 30 minutes a day, or 45 minutes two or three times a week.

Cycling, Trampolining, Going to the Gym, or Jogging

Your aim is the same as for walking or swimming. Start with a short easy routine—10 to 15 minutes per day, and slowly work up to about 30 minutes a day. Gradually increase your work rate without ever straining yourself.

Apart from the fact that jumping up and down makes you feel like a kid again, trampolining causes every cell in the body to respond. Balance, reflexes, and circulation improve, your colon is stimulated, body toned, muscles strengthened, and feet massaged.

When I go to the gym I sometimes see people spending untold minutes and hours on one machine. If you go to the gym, vary the exercises. For example, do 10 minutes on the treadmill, 10 minutes on the stairs, 10 minutes of lifting weights, and so on. This way, you vary your workout, don't get bored, and get all the benefits.

If jogging, please invest in a good pair of running shoes that offer cushioned support, and if you're a woman, for all activities invest in a good sports bra.

Is There Anything I Should Do before and after I Exercise?

► Make sure that you drink adequate fluids in advance of your exercise; otherwise you run the risk of becoming dehydrated and ending up with a headache.

► Start an exercise session with a gradual warm-up period. During this time (about 5 to 10 minutes), you should slowly stretch your muscles first and then gradually increase your level of activity. For example, begin walking slowly and then pick up the pace.

► After you are finished exercising, cool down for about 5 to 10 minutes. If you have been jogging, slow down to a gentle walk before stopping. You are stretching your muscles and allowing your heart rate to slow down gradually. You can use the same stretches as in the warm-up period.

HOW HARD DO I HAVE TO EXERCISE?

Even small amounts of exercise are better than none at all. Start with an activity you can do comfortably. As a rule of thumb, when you are exercising you should be slightly out of breath but not so out of breath that you can't hold a conversation with someone. So if you find yourself panting, huffing, and puffing within a few minutes, stop. You're exercising too hard.

HOW DO I STAY MOTIVATED?

FIND A FITNESS PARTNER Find a walking partner, play tennis with your spouse or a friend, or go rollerblading with the kids.

SCHEDULE YOUR WORKOUTS Exercise must be a priority in order to establish it as a lifestyle practice. Make time for your workouts and schedule them on your daily calendar or planner.

DRESS THE PART Wear comfortable clothes appropriate for exercising. They will help you feel like working out. If you exercise at a gym, put your exercise wear in a bag and set it beside the door the night before. When it's time to head out the door, all you have to do is grab your bag on the way out.

ENTERTAIN YOURSELF If you exercise alone, consider using a portable music device to listen to your favorite music or books on tape to help keep you entertained during your workout. Many pieces of exercise equipment have racks that fit onto the console to hold reading material. If you exercise at home, turn on some music or bring the television within viewing range.

MAKE EXERCISE NON-NEGOTIABLE Think of exercise as something you do without question, like brushing your teeth or going to work. Taking this lifestyle perspective will help you make exercise a habit.
WARNING! NEVER OVERDO EXERCISE!

DR. GILLIAN'S FAT FLUSH

FAT FLUSH FOR WEIGHT LOSS

If you are overweight, you could get
your plan started with my two-day detox
followed by the Fat Flush day. This will
help cleanse your system and make the
28-day plan even more effective.

BREAKFAST

**A cup of warm water with a squeeze
of lemon and lime
Two whole pink grapefruit**

LUNCH
Mung Bean Casserole with Special Brown Rice

Mung Bean Casserole
SERVES 2
**4¹/₂ oz. mung beans
2¹/₈ cups water or vegetable stock
   plus water to soak
1 tsp fennel seeds
1 onion, finely chopped
2 carrots, peeled and diced
2 tbsps flat leaf parsley, chopped
1 endive
handful clover sprouts**

1. Soak the mung beans in 1 quart of cold
water for 6 hours. Drain and rinse well.
Bring the water or stock to a boil, add the
beans, and simmer for 10 minutes. Skim away
any white scum that rises to the surface.
2. Add the fennel seeds and simmer for
10 minutes. Then add the onion and carrots
and simmer for an additional 10 minutes.
3. Remove from heat and add the parsley.
4. Arrange the endive leaves around the edge
of two soup bowls, pour the casserole into the
center of the bowls, sprinkle over the clover
sprouts, and serve with Special Brown Rice.

Special Brown Rice
**3¹/₂ oz. brown rice
1 onion, peeled and chopped
⁷/₈ cup water
¹/₂ tsp turmeric
¹/₂ tsp cumin**

1. Place the rice, spices, and onion in a
saucepan. Add water.
2. Bring the water to a boil, lower heat,
and simmer for 20 minutes.
3. Turn off the heat, and allow to stand
for 10 minutes before serving.

DINNER
Chilled Cucumber Soup with Coleslaw Salad

Chilled Cucumber Soup
SERVES 2
3 cucumbers
4 scallions, finely sliced
2 1/8 cups water
juice of half a lemon
6–8 mint leaves
1 3/4 oz. sprouting beans

1. Cut one cucumber in half and finely dice. Reserve for the garnish.
2. Take the remaining cucumbers, peel, halve, and with a teaspoon remove the seeds and discard.
3. Place the deseeded cucumbers in a food processor with the scallions and water, and blend until smooth.
4. Add the lemon juice and mint leaves and blend again.
5. Put into bowls and chill well. Serve with sprouting beans and diced cucumber sprinkled over the top.

Coleslaw Salad
1 carrot trimmed
1 scallion
1 1/4 oz. walnut pieces
small piece of white cabbage, cored
   and shredded
1 celery stalk
1 tbsp chopped cilantro or chopped parsley
1/2 oz. fresh garden peas
3 radishes, finely chopped
FOR THE DRESSING, BLEND THE FOLLOWING:
4 tbsps hemp oil
1 handful arugula leaves
2 tbsps pine nuts
1 garlic clove, peeled and crushed

EVENING
Mix 7/8 cup of pink grapefruit juice and 2 tbsps of olive oil or hemp oil and drink.

Drink warm cups of water throughout the day. Alternate between sage tea and an herbal tea called Pau d'arco tea during the day (available from health food stores).

the plan

Day 1

BREAKFAST

1 cup of warm water with a squeeze of lemon
1 cup nettle tea
followed by fruit salad and a bowl
of quick oats.

Fruit Berry Salad
SERVES 1
1 small tub blueberries
1 small tub raspberries
1 small basket strawberries

Quick Oats
If you are still hungry, you can have
a bowl of oats, but you need to
wait 20 minutes to let your fruit digest.

SERVES 1
3¹/₂ oz. oats
1²/₃ cups water or rice milk

1. Combine the oats with water or rice milk in
a pan.
2. Bring to a boil, then lower the heat
and simmer for 15–20 minutes.
3. Season with a sprinkle of cinnamon.

MID-MORNING SNACK
Veggie Juice or two celery stalks with dip
(see page 200 for dips).

Veggie Juice
SERVES 1
2 celery stalks
6 carrots

LUNCH

Tuna and Leafy Salad
SERVES 1
1 small bag watercress,
   spinach, and arugula salad
7-oz. can tuna steak in spring water
handful of halved cherry tomatoes
a few slices cucumber
1–2 tbsp chopped, fresh dill
squeeze of lemon juice

1. Shake the bag of leaf salad into a bowl.
2. Top with the drained can of tuna steak.
Flake into chunks with a fork.
3. Add the halved cherry tomatoes,
cucumber, and dill.
4. Drizzle with freshly squeezed lemon
juice before serving.

MID-AFTERNOON SNACK
Veggie Juice or one whole yellow pepper, finely chopped.

Veggie Juice
SERVES 1
6 celery stalks
1 cucumber
1 yellow pepper

DINNER

Poached Chicken in Ginger Miso with Bok Choy

SERVES 1

1 free range chicken breast
1¼ cups vegetable stock or make
  stock with a veggie cube
1 tbsp organic miso
½–¾" piece of fresh ginger
2 cloves garlic, peeled and chopped
3 tbsps fresh cilantro
½ red pepper, finely sliced
1 handful beansprouts
2 bok choy trimmed and roughly
  chopped, save 2 leaves for garnish

1. Preheat oven to 390°F. Take a large sheet of foil and place the chicken in the center.
2. In a small pan, bring the stock to a boil and add the miso, ginger, garlic, and 1 tbsp of the cilantro.
3. Pull the foil up to create a bowl shape and spoon over the flavored stock. Scrunch the foil up to create a parcel. Transfer to a baking tray and cook for 10 minutes.
4. Arrange the bok choy on a serving plate. Transfer the cooked chicken onto the bok choy and then sprinkle over the pepper and sprouts.
5. Garnish with the two whole leaves of bok choy and remaining cilantro. Serve immediately.

VEGETARIAN ALTERNATIVE
Marinated Veggie Tofu

SERVES 2

6¼ oz. chilled tofu, cut into ½" cubes
1 medium carrot, sliced
1 red pepper, sliced
2½ oz. sugar snap peas
2 oz. broccoli florets
¾ oz. cashews
2 scallions, finely sliced
FOR THE MARINADE
2 tbsps wheat-free tamari sauce
1 garlic clove, peeled and crushed
1 tsp finely chopped fresh root ginger

1. Mix the marinade in a shallow dish and marinate the tofu for 10 minutes.
2. Stir-fry the carrot, pepper, sugar snap peas, and broccoli with cold pressed sunflower oil and a little water, for 3 minutes.
3. Lift the tofu out of the marinade with a slotted spoon and add to the pan with the cashew nuts and scallions.
4. Stir-fry for 1–2 minutes, turning gently until the tofu is hot.

Drink a cup of warm water an hour before bed every day of the Plan.

Day 2

BREAKFAST

1 cup of warm water
1 cup dandelion tea
followed by a smoothie.

Peach and Mango Smoothie
SERVES 1
1 large mango, stoned and chopped
1 peach, stoned and chopped
1 banana, sliced
1 cup water
1 small tub blueberries

1. Blend all ingredients
(except blueberries) until smooth.
2. Add more water if you want
a thinner consistency.
3. Pour over the blueberries and drink.

MID-MORNING SNACK
Bowl of grapes.

LUNCH
Miso Soup followed by Avocado and Pine Nut Salad.

Miso Soup
Simply add miso powder to a mug of water
and drink. There are different flavors of miso,
and some miso packs come with tofu added
too. So easy.

Avocado and Pine Nut Salad
SERVES 2
2 little gem lettuces
1 avocado
4 tomatoes, quartered
1 red pepper, sliced
1 yellow pepper, sliced
handful of fresh basil leaves
handful of alfalfa sprouts (optional)
handful of radishes (optional)
2 tbsps extra virgin olive oil or hemp oil
3 tbsps pine nuts

1. Separate and wash the lettuce leaves.
2. Place the lettuce in a large bowl with the
avocado, tomatoes, peppers, and basil leaves.
3. If possible add a generous serving of
alfalfa sprouts and decorate with a handful
of radishes.
4. Drizzle with 2 tbsps of extra virgin olive
oil or hemp oil and sprinkle with 2–3 tbsps
pine nuts.

MID-AFTERNOON SNACK
**Cucumber and carrot crudités with hummus,
sprinkled with dill.**

Keep smelling sweet from your insides
with a mango. Mango acts like an
internal deodorant because it contains
antioxidants that can help eliminate
odor-causing bacteria.

DINNER

Poached Monkfish with Tarragon

You can use any firm, white fish, but monkfish is particularly good. With all the recipes, don't fret if you can't find a particular ingredient, I just want to give you lots of ideas.

SERVES 2
5 oz. baby spinach leaves
2 vine ripened tomatoes, sliced
2 cups water
1 bay leaf
1/2–3/4" piece fresh ginger, peeled
1 lemongrass stalk
2 cloves garlic, peeled
1 Kaffir lime leaf, or juice of lime
1 tsp fresh miso paste
7 oz. piece fresh monkfish
large handful fresh tarragon
1 tsp olive oil

1. Arrange the baby spinach and tomatoes on a serving plate.
2. Bring the water to a boil with the bay leaf, ginger, lemongrass, garlic, Kaffir lime leaf, and miso paste. Boil for 5 minutes and then reduce to a simmer.
3. Poach the fish for 3–4 minutes or until firm to the touch.
4. Remove the fish from the pan and keep it warm while you finish the sauce.
5. Boil the liquid until the volume has reduced by half.
6. Remove from heat and strain in a small bowl, discarding the seasoning.
7. Add the tarragon and oil, and with a hand-held blender blitz until smooth. Alternatively this can be done in a small processor.
8. Place the fish on the spinach and tomatoes, spoon over the sauce, and serve.

Day 3

BREAKFAST

1 cup of warm water with a squeeze of lemon
1 cup nettle tea
followed by a smoothie.

Strawberry Smoothie
SERVES 1
1 small basket strawberries, hulled
$1/2$ small tub raspberries
2 ripe pears, cored and chopped
1 apple, peeled and chopped
1 cup water

Blend all the ingredients until smooth.

MID-MORNING SNACK
**Four endive leaves, topped with hummus
and baby tomatoes.**

LUNCH
**Baked Sweet Potato with sprouted alfalfa seeds
and a Beet Salad.**

Sweet Potato
Pop a large sweet potato into the oven for
30 minutes while you prepare your salad.

Beet Salad
Baby beets are best for this salad, but you
can use larger beets and peel them before
making the salad.

SERVES 1
18 oz. baby beets
1 tbsp cider vinegar
$1/2$ cucumber, finely sliced
1 tbsp sesame seeds
2 tbsps alfalfa sprouts

1. Scrub the beets well and trim the stalks to
about $1-1^{1/2}$" in length and then place in
a steamer and cook for 7–10 minutes. The
time will depend on the size of the beets.
2. Allow the beets to cool slightly, then
cut in half and arrange on a serving plate
with the cucumber.
3. Pour over the vinegar, sprinkle with the
sesame seeds and alfalfa sprouts, and serve.

MID-AFTERNOON SNACK
**Veggie Juice or a handful of salt-free organic almonds
(if you can soak the almonds first in water they will be
even easier to digest).**

Veggie Juice
SERVES 1
4 carrots
$1/2$ beet
2 celery stalks

DINNER
Soup with Lemon and Fennel Coleslaw.

White Bean Soup

My creamy white bean soup is perfect if you miss soups with cream in them. Coriander seeds are available in health food shops and can be ground in a clean pepper grinder. Reserve a portion for lunch tomorrow.

SERVES 4
1 onion, peeled and chopped
2 leeks, sliced
2 cloves garlic, peeled and chopped
1 tsp olive oil
2 cups vegetable stock or water
2 bay leaves
small bunch parsley stalks
freshly ground coriander seeds
16-oz. can cannelini beans, drained
fresh chives to garnish

1. Place the onion, leeks, garlic, oil, and a little water in a medium-sized pan. Cook over moderate heat for 5 minutes until the vegetables are slightly softened. Do not allow the vegetables to color.
2. Bring the vegetable stock to a boil and pour over the vegetables. Add the bay leaves and parsley. Season with the coriander seeds.
3. Return the soup to a boil and simmer for 15 minutes.
4. Add the beans for 3–4 minutes on a very low heat until they are warmed through.
5. Remove the pan from the heat and allow to cool slightly. Remove the bay leaf, then blend with a stick blender or in the food processor.
6. Spoon into warmed deep soup bowls. Sprinkle with fresh chives and serve immediately.

SERVES 2
12 1/2 oz. red cabbage
1 fennel bulb, trimmed and finely sliced
2 celery sticks, trimmed and sliced
2 scallions, trimmed and sliced
4 tbsps freshly squeezed lemon juice
3 tbsps extra virgin olive oil
1 3/4 oz. walnut halves, roughly chopped

1. Remove the outer leaves of the cabbage and cut out and discard the central core.
2. Slice the cabbage very finely and place in a serving bowl—you should have around 9 3/4 oz. prepared weight.
3. Add the fennel, celery, scallions, lemon juice, and oil. Toss well together and sprinkle with the walnuts just before serving.

Fennel removes fat and mucus from the intestinal tract and acts like a natural appetite suppressant.

Day 4

BREAKFAST

1 cup of warm water
1 cup dandelion tea
followed by fruit salad and Savory Quinoa.

Fruit Salad
1 apple
1 pear
1 peach
2 apricots

Savory Quinoa
Use the grain, not the flakes. Remember
to allow 20 minutes between eating your
fruit and your porridge. If you are in a rush,
pour the quinoa into a container and take
it to work.

SERVES 1–2
5¼ oz. quinoa
1½ cups water
2 tsps sesame seeds
dried mixed herbs (optional)

1. Put the quinoa and water in a pan.
Bring to boil and simmer for 8 minutes.
2. Allow the porridge to sit for a few
minutes and serve.
3. Garnish with dried mixed herbs if you
need extra flavor.

MID-MORNING SNACK
Juice of two whole pink grapefruit.

LUNCH
White Bean Soup from the night before, with Zesty
Avocado Mayo served with vegetable crudités (raw veggies
chopped in strips or bite-sized chunks for dipping).

Zesty Avocado Mayo
It keeps well in the fridge for 24 hours.

SERVES 2
1 ripe avocado
½ tsp finely grated lemon zest
2 tbsps freshly squeezed lemon juice

1. Blend all the ingredients together using
a stick blender until smooth and creamy
(or mash very well with a fork). Add a little
more lemon juice if desired.
2. Spoon into a small dish and cover the
surface tightly with non-PVC cling wrap
to prevent browning.
3. Chill until ready to serve.

MID-AFTERNOON SNACK
Bowl of cherries.

DINNER

Adzuki Bean Bake with savoy cabbage, green beans, or broccoli.

It's that time again. Ah yes. It's time for the adzuki beans! You cannot escape adzuki beans à la Dr. Gillian! But this new recipe is a whole new way to get these healthy beans into you.

Adzuki Bean Bake

This recipe makes two generous servings, so save some for the next day's lunch.

SERVES 2

1 tbsp olive oil, plus extra for brushing
1 medium onion, peeled and chopped
2 garlic cloves, peeled and crushed
1 small squash, peeled and diced
1 large carrot, peeled and diced
1 celery stick, trimmed and sliced
2 cups just-boiled water
1 tsp organic vegetable bouillon
   (stock) powder
5³/4 oz. cooked adzuki beans
1 medium leek, trimmed and sliced
2 tsps cornstarch or arrowroot blended with
1 tbsp cold water to make a smooth paste
1 large sweet potato, cut into ¹/8" slices
(If you like a lot of topping, use 2 potatoes.)

1. Heat the oil in a large saucepan with a tiny bit of water, so you are water sautéing really. You are not frying in the normal sense of the word.
2. Gently water sauté the onion and garlic for 3 minutes, stirring occasionally.
3. Add the squash, carrot, and celery. Cook with the onion and garlic for 2 minutes, stirring regularly.
4. Pour the just-boiled water over the vegetables and stir in the bouillon powder.
5. Bring to a boil, then reduce the heat and simmer for 10 minutes.
6. Preheat the oven to 390°F.
7. Stir the sliced leek and adzuki beans into the vegetable mixture. Return to a simmer and cook for 5 minutes, stirring occasionally.
8. Add the cornflour or arrowroot mixture and cook for about 1 minute until the sauce thickens, stirring.
9. Remove from the heat and transfer carefully into a 3 ³/4 cup ovenproof dish.
10. Arrange slices of the sweet potato on top of the bean and vegetable mixture. Brush with a little of the oil and bake for about 30 minutes until the potato is soft.
11. Serve with freshly cooked savoy cabbage, green beans, or broccoli and raw snow peas.

Hail to the Adzuki Bean, my Bean of Weight Loss. Packed with weight-regulating nutrients, adzuki beans act like a sponge soaking up excess fluid in the body. Adzukis are my bean of choice for you for weight loss. Eat them at least once a week.

Day 5

BREAKFAST

1 cup of warm water with a squeeze of lemon
1 cup slippery elm tea
followed by vegetable juice.

Ginger Zinger
If you are running late, pour the juice into
a container with a straw and drink it on
the way.

SERVES 1
6 carrots
1/2 tsp chopped ginger
1 cucumber
1 stick of celery

1. Push all the ingredients through the
funnel of the juicer and pour into a glass.
2. Sip slowly.

REMEMBER TO LEAVE YOUR YELLOW SPLIT PEAS TO
SOAK IN PLENTY OF WATER TO READY FOR THE
EVENING.

MID-MORNING SNACK
Two peaches.

LUNCH
Adzuki Bean Bake from last night, heat and serve on a bed
of raw leaves, herbs, and sprouted seeds of your choice.

MID-AFTERNOON SNACK
Veggie Juice or one fennel bulb, chopped and served
with a dip (see page 200 for dips).

Veggie Juice
SERVES 1
1 fennel
1/2 beet
1 cucumber

DINNER
Soup and Oriental Style Salad.

Easy Peasy Yellow Pea Soup
Save a portion for lunch tomorrow.

SERVES 4
8 oz. yellow split peas, soaked for 3 hours
1 sweet potato
2 carrots
2 onions
1 tbsp salt-free bouillon powder

1. Sieve the peas and rinse well under cold water. Put them in a pan with 1 1/2 qt. water.
2. Bring to a boil and skim off the excess foam.
3. Add the sweet potato, carrots, onion, and bouillon.
4. Boil for 10 minutes, lower the heat, then simmer for another 15 minutes.
5. Blend until smooth, or blend half of the soup, then mix it back in with the half you didn't blend—this makes it more chunky.
6. Pour into warmed bowls, toss a handful of fresh, raw alfalfa sprouts into each bowl, and serve immediately.

Oriental Style Salad
SERVES 1
1 zucchini
1/2 cucumber
1/2 red or yellow pepper
1 carrot
2 scallions, sliced
beansprouts
green salad leaves
FOR THE DRESSING
1 tbsp wheat-free tamari sauce
1 tsp sesame oil
2 tbsps water
1 clove garlic, crushed

1. Cut the zucchini, cucumber, peppers, and carrots into long thin sticks.
2. Toss with sliced scallions and rinsed beansprouts.
3. Mix together tamari sauce, sesame oil, water, and garlic.
4. Drizzle the dressing over the salad.
5. Serve over green salad leaves.

Cucumbers are a fabulous food for weight loss and a perfect anti-bloat food because of their diuretic properties. So don't scoff at them, just eat them and make lots of juices with them too.

Day 6

BREAKFAST

1 cup of warm water with a squeeze of lemon
1 cup of dandelion tea
followed by a smoothie.

Plummy Fruit Smoothie
This smoothie is also delicious with
a few berries added to the blend.

SERVES 1
3 plums
3 nectarines
3 ripe pears
1 cup water

Blend all ingredients until smooth
and creamy.

REMEMBER TO SOAK YOUR MUNG BEANS
FOR DINNER TONIGHT.

MID-MORNING SNACK
One ripe banana.

LUNCH

**Easy Peasy Yellow Pea Soup (from
last night) with Avocado and Salad.**
Sprinkle your soup with raw shelled hemp
seeds and/or sprouted alfalfa seeds.

Avocado
One ripe avocado, halved and stoned.

**Purple Sprouting Broccoli Salad
with Radish**
The pistachio nuts add a lovely crunch
to this salad, but if you are seriously trying
for weight loss, then I would advise that
you omit them at this time.

SERVES 1
2$\frac{1}{2}$ oz. well-trimmed purple sprouting broccoli
1 oz. fresh radish, sliced
1 oz. shelled peas
$\frac{1}{2}$ tbsp mirin
1$\frac{1}{2}$ tbsps wheat-free tamari sauce
1 tbsp pistachio nuts (optional)

1. Cut the broccoli in half lengthways and
then into bite-sized pieces, then arrange
on a salad plate.
2. Scatter over the radish and peas, then
sprinkle with the mirin and tamari.
3. Add the nuts and serve immediately.

MID-AFTERNOON SNACK
**Four endive leaves, topped with hummus
and baby tomatoes.**

DINNER
Gourmet Mighty Mung Bean Casserole served with brown rice and salad.

Gourmet Mighty Mung Bean Casserole
Reserve a portion for your lunch tomorrow.

SERVES 4–6
**8 3/4 oz. mung beans, soaked in 1 qt. cold
    water for 6 hours
1 qt. water or vegetable stock
1 tsp fennel seeds
6 1/4 oz. celeriac, peeled and diced
3 1/2 oz. celery, chopped
5 1/4 oz. leeks, chopped
2 small bok choy
watercress or arugula**

1. Drain the mung beans and rinse well.
2. Bring the water or stock to a boil,
add the beans, and simmer for 10 minutes.
Skim away any white scum that rises
to the surface.
3. Add the fennel seeds and celeriac and
simmer for 10 minutes.
4. Add the celery and leeks and simmer
for 10 more minutes.
5. Remove from heat. Stir in the bok choy, put
in warmed bowls, and sprinkle with the
watercress or arugula.
6. Serve with a simple green leafy salad
and brown rice.

The Mighty Mung Bean—my antitoxin. I rave about the mung bean, as many of you probably know. They cook very quickly and are super easy to digest. I use mung beans to purge the body of toxins or excess acids caused by poor diets. And mung beans release energy steadily, keeping blood sugar balanced.

Day 7

BREAKFAST

1 cup of warm water with squeeze of lemon
1 cup of dandelion tea
followed by a smoothie.

Tangy Smoothie
SERVES 1
1/2 **pineapple**
1 mango
1 banana
1 plum

Blend all ingredients until smooth
and creamy.

MID-MORNING SNACK
One or more apples.

LUNCH
Mung Bean Salad made from Gourmet Mighty
Mung Bean Casserole.

Mung Bean Salad
SERVES 1
1 portion of Gourmet Mighty Mung Bean
   Casserole, and any leftover brown rice
2 oz. radish
3 scallions
1 tbsp lemon juice
1³/4 oz. fresh arugula
2 tbsps raw shelled hemp seeds (optional)

1. Drain any excess moisture from the beans.
2. Place in a mixing bowl with all the other
ingredients and toss them together.
3. Serve immediately.

MID-AFTERNOON SNACK
Veggie Juice or a handful of salt-free hazelnuts
(organic if possible).

Veggie Juice
SERVES 1
handful of spinach
6 carrots
3 celery stalks

DINNER
Baked Whitefish with Minted Mushy Peas on a bed of salad.

Baked Whitefish with Minted Mushy Peas

Any whitefish works well in this recipe, whiting, haddock, or cod, for example. This is a great fast meal to make when you get in from work.

SERVES 4
1 tsp oil
4 3½-oz. skinless whitefish fillets
1 lemon, sliced
2 cloves garlic, peeled and sliced
a few sprigs of dill or fennel
4½ oz. new season or frozen peas
a large sprig of fresh mint
1 tsp mirin

1. Preheat the oven to 390°F.
2. Take a large piece of foil and, with a pastry brush, oil the center. Place the fish on the foil and cover with the lemon slices and garlic. Scatter over the dill or fennel. Scrunch up the foil to make a parcel and place on a baking tray.

3. Place in the oven and cook for 6–7 minutes. Remove from the oven and allow to stand for 10 minutes.
4. Bring a small pan of water to a boil and add the mint and peas and cook (fresh peas for 1–2 minutes, frozen for 30 seconds). Remove from heat and drain.
5. Place the peas in a small bowl with the mirin and mash with a fork.
6. Divide the peas and fish between four warmed serving plates and serve immediately with some raw green salad leaves.

SOAK 1 CUP OF BUCKWHEAT OVERNIGHT FOR YOUR MORNING PORRIDGE. THIS WAY YOUR PORRIDGE WILL BE READY IN NO TIME.

Look at yourself in a mirror right now. See and envision the possibilities of who you can truly be when you set your mind to it.

Day 8

1 cup of warm water
1 cup of dandelion tea
followed by 1 large grapefruit and Buckwheat
Cinnamon Porridge.

Buckwheat Cinnamon Porridge
SERVES 1–2
4¹/₂ oz. buckwheat groats
1 tsp lemon zest and a squeeze of lemon juice
¹/₂" piece fresh ginger root, peeled and grated
1 cinnamon stick, broken
raw shelled hemp seeds or sunflower seeds
   (optional)

1. Place the buckwheat, lemon zest and
juice, ginger, cinnamon, and 2 cups of water
in a pan. Bring to a boil, then lower the heat
and simmer for 20 minutes.
2. Serve with a sprinkling of sunflower
or shelled hemp seeds.

MID-MORNING SNACK
Small baskets of berries (choose from strawberries,
gooseberries, blackberries, or blueberries).

My dad introduced me
to grapefruit for breakfast
as a child. I am glad he
was a grapefruit fanatic
as they are packed with
antioxidants.

LUNCH
Navy Bean Salad.

Navy Bean Salad
SERVES 2
1 can no salt, no sugar navy beans
1/2 red onion, finely chopped
1 clove garlic, crushed
1 tbsp fresh parsley, chopped
2 tbsps extra virgin olive oil
2 tsps apple cider vinegar
1 small bag mixed leaf and herb salad
1 endive, sliced
1 red pepper, finely diced
8–10 green beans

1. Drain the navy beans and rinse
under cold water.
2. Put the beans, red onion, garlic, parsley,
olive oil, and cider vinegar in a bowl, toss
together, then set aside for 10 minutes.
3. Cook the green beans in boiling water
for 2–3 minutes, then plunge into cold
water to cool.
4. Empty the mixed leaf and herb salad into
a bowl. Add the endive, red pepper, and cooled
green beans.
5. Spoon the navy beans with dressing over
the salad and serve.

MID-AFTERNOON SNACK
Vegetable crudités (four radishes and one
yellow pepper, chopped) and dip (see page 200
for dips).

DINNER
**Fresh vegetable juice followed by baked squash with
mashed avocado and beansprout topping.**

Veggie Juice
C'mon, you can do it. It'll take you two
minutes. If you don't manage a veggie juice
during the day, it's a fantastic pick-me-up
for when you come home from work.

SERVES 1
4–5 carrots
1 cucumber
1 stick of celery

Juice all ingredients and drink slowly.

Baked Squash
Pop a squash in the oven and let it bake
while you drink your juice.

Topping
You can add any fresh raw vegetables
to this mix, just mash them all in there.

SERVES 1
1 avocado
fresh dill
generous portion of beansprouts
generous portion of alfalfa sprouts
2 radishes, sliced
lemon juice

1. Mash the avocado with the dill,
beansprouts, and alfalfa sprouts.
2. Squeeze some lemon juice over the top
and add a couple of radishes for garnish.
3. Pile on top of baked squash and serve.

Day 9

BREAKFAST

1 cup of warm water
1 cup of dandelion tea
followed by fruit salad.

Fruit Salad
SERVES 1
1 banana
1/2 small tub blueberries
1 peach
1/2 small tub raspberries or strawberries

MID-MORNING SNACK
A cup of instant miso soup. Add four chopped radishes for a crunchy texture.

LUNCH
Risotto of Fennel and Fava Beans.

Risotto of Fennel and Fava Beans
SERVES 1
1 small onion, finely chopped
1/2 fennel bulb, core removed, finely chopped
2 cloves garlic, chopped
2 tsps olive oil
1 tbsp water
3 1/2 oz. brown rice
1 cup vegetable stock
2 3/4 oz. baby fava beans
2 tbsps freshly chopped chervil

1. Place the onion, fennel, garlic, oil, and water in a non-stick pan and cook gently for 5 minutes.
2. Add the rice and stir well.
3. Gradually add the stock, 1 ladleful at a time, and cook until the rice is tender—about 15–20 minutes.
4. Stir in the fava beans and chervil and serve immediately.

MID-AFTERNOON SNACK
Small bowl of cherry tomatoes or baby plum tomatoes.

Miso is one of the most valuable healing foods, and I want you to try it. It's made from fermented soybean paste, and it has a unique nutritional profile packed with easily digestable protein and energy-boosting vitamins. You can find it in powder or paste form in the health food store. Use miso in your cooking instead of plain old table salt and reap a variety of benefits in addition to enhanced flavor.

DINNER

Soup, followed by Baked Salmon served with steamed vegetables.

5 Minute Soup

Save a portion for your lunch tomorrow.

SERVES 1–2
2 cups water
1 clove garlic
small piece of fresh root ginger, peeled
   and finely sliced
4 oz. slab of firm tofu, cut into small
   squares
8 snow peas, trimmed and finely sliced
   lengthways
1 small red pepper, de-seeded and cut
   into short thin strips
small handful of fresh or frozen peas
1 bok choy, leaves separated, washed
   and sliced
2 scallions, trimmed and sliced
2 sachets of instant miso soup
   (robust flavor)
handful of alfalfa sprouts
fresh cilantro to garnish

1. Bring the water to a boil in a large
saucepan, add the garlic and ginger, and
boil for 1 minute.
2. Stir in the tofu, snow peas, pepper, and
peas. Return to a boil, skim any foam from
the surface with a spoon, and simmer for
2 minutes.
3. Add the bok choy and scallions
and cook for 1 minute.
4. Remove from the heat and stir in the
miso soup and beansprouts.
5. Ladle into a warmed bowl to serve.
Garnish with fresh chopped cilantro.

Simple Baked Salmon

SERVES 1
boneless fillet of salmon
small head of broccoli
2 carrots, cut into batons
lemon and lime wedges to serve
salad leaves (optional)

1. Heat the oven to 390°F.
2. Place the salmon on a baking tray and
cook in the oven for 18–20 minutes until
cooked through.
3. Steam the carrots for a few minutes,
then add the broccoli and lightly cook.
4. Place the carrots and broccoli on a plate
and lay the salmon fillet on top. Add a couple
of lime and lemon wedges for squeezing
over the fish.
5. Serve with some raw salad leaves
if you like.

**PUT 3 ½ OZ. ADZUKI BEANS IN A BOWL WITH PLENTY OF
COLD WATER AND LEAVE THEM IN THE FRIDGE TO SOAK
OVERNIGHT (FOR DINNER TOMORROW).**

Day 10

BREAKFAST

1 cup of warm water
1 cup fennel tea
followed by Stewed Apples.

Stewed Apples over Fresh Blueberries

Fresh raspberries also work well with stewed apple.

SERVES 1
2 apples
1 cup water
squeeze of lemon juice
1 pear, chopped
1 tub blueberries

1. Chop the apples, put them in a pan with the water and lemon juice, and stew until soft.
2. Serve over the chopped pear and blueberries.

MID-MORNING SNACK

Two papayas or two nectarines.

LUNCH

5 Minute Soup from yesterday, followed by Fresh Tuna with Steamed Kale and Caper Dressing.

Fresh Tuna with Steamed Kale and Caper Dressing

In this recipe you could use crushed chickpeas flavored with a little brown rice vinegar instead of the avocado, and use parsley rather than capers.

SERVES 1
5 oz. tuna steak
5 oz. fresh kale
1 avocado, peeled and with pit removed
FOR THE DRESSING
3 tbsps capers
2–3 tbsps fresh parsley
juice of 1 lemon, plus a little extra
1 tsp oil
3 tbsps hot water

1. Heat a non-stick pan and cook the tuna for 2–3 minutes on each side.
2. Remove the tuna from the pan. Add the kale to the pan with 1 tbsp water and cook for 2 minutes, or until just wilted.
3. Mix the capers, parsley, lemon juice, oil, and hot water together and whisk well.
4. Crush the avocado with a little lemon juice, using the back of a fork.
5. Place the avocado on a serving plate and arrange the kale around it. Place the tuna on the avocado.
6. Spoon over half the dressing (reserve the rest for a salad tomorrow) and serve immediately.

MID-AFTERNOON SNACK
Veggie Juice or half a cucumber, finely chopped.

Veggie Juice
SERVES 1
1 cucumber
2 celery stalks
handful alfalfa sprouts
tiny piece of ginger

DINNER
Adzuki Bean Hotpot served with Crunchy Green Salad.

Adzuki Bean Hotpot
The fresher the beans, the quicker they
will cook, but there is no way of telling
how fresh they are when you buy them.
So be prepared to cook the beans for longer
if necessary and add extra water if they
appear to be drying out. Reserve a portion
for your lunch tomorrow.

SERVES 4
3$^{1}/_{2}$ oz. dried adzuki beans, soaked and rinsed
2 qt. cold water
1 tbsp extra virgin olive oil
1 medium onion, peeled and chopped
2 garlic cloves, peeled and crushed
1 celery stick, trimmed and sliced
3 medium carrots, peeled and sliced
1 large parsnip, peeled and cubed
1 large sweet potato, peeled and cubed
    (around 14 oz. prepared weight)
14-oz. can chopped tomatoes
$^{1}/_{2}$ organic wheat-free stock cube
2 medium leeks, trimmed and sliced

1. Place the beans in a bowl to soak, cover with plenty of cold water, and leave in the fridge overnight. Drain well.

2. Place the soaked beans in a large saucepan. Cover with 2 qt. cold water and bring to a boil. Boil hard for 15 minutes, then reduce the heat slightly and simmer for a further 30–40 minutes until the beans are tender, stirring occasionally. Add an extra cup or two of water if the beans begin to look dry.

3. While the beans are cooking, heat the oil in a large saucepan or flame-proof casserole and very gently cook the onion, garlic, and celery for 5 minutes until well softened but not colored, stirring regularly.

4. Add the carrots, parsnip, and sweet potato to the pan. Cook gently for 10 minutes, stirring occasionally.

5. Stir in the canned tomatoes. Fill half of the empty can with water and pour over the vegetables.

6. Add the half stock cube and bring to a boil. Reduce the heat slightly and simmer for 5 minutes.

7. Add the leeks and continue to simmer for 10–15 minutes more until all the vegetables are just tender and the sauce is thick.

8. Drain the cooked adzuki beans in a colander and stir into the vegetable mixture.

9. Spoon the adzuki bean mixture into a 2 qt. ovenproof dish. Bake in a preheated oven at 390°F for 20 minutes.

10. Serve with Crunchy Green Salad.

Crunchy Green Salad

SERVES 3–4

1 large handful fine green beans, trimmed
5 oz. asparagus tips, trimmed
5 oz. tenderstem broccoli, trimmed and broken into thin lengths
4 tbsps fresh or frozen peas
1 fennel bulb, trimmed and finely sliced
2 celery sticks, trimmed and sliced
1 little gem lettuce, trimmed and thickly sliced
3 tbsps pine nuts
3 tbsps pumpkin seeds
FOR THE DRESSING
4 tbsps extra virgin olive oil
1 tbsp freshly squeezed lemon juice
1 garlic clove, peeled and crushed

1. Bring a large pan of water to a boil. Add the green beans, return to a boil, and cook for 2 minutes.

2. Add the asparagus, tenderstem broccoli, and peas. Return to a boil and cook for just 1 minute. Drain the beans and asparagus in a colander and rinse under running water until cold. Transfer to a serving dish.

3. Toss the fennel, celery, little gem lettuce, pine nuts, and pumpkin seeds with the blanched vegetables.

4. Whisk the oil, lemon juice, and garlic together with a fork and pour over the salad just before serving.

Day 11

BREAKFAST

1 cup of warm water
1 cup slippery elm tea
followed by fruit salad.

Fruit Salad
SERVES 1
1 apple
2 peaches
1 pear
1 banana

MID-MORNING SNACK
Juice of two whole pink grapefruit.

LUNCH
Adzuki Bean Hotpot from yesterday, served with salad.

Snow Pea and Sauerkraut Salad
SERVES 1
6 snow peas
4 endive leaves
1 tbsp sauerkraut
1 little gem lettuce, shredded
squeeze of lemon juice
2 tsps hemp oil
2 lightly steamed asparagus (optional),
   finely chopped

1. Arrange the raw ingredients in an artistic
way on a large plate.
2. Drizzle the hemp oil over the salad and top
with a squeeze of lemon and the asparagus.

MID-AFTERNOON SNACK
Handful of unsalted cashews and handful
of sunflower/pumpkin seeds.

DINNER
Soup followed by Butter Bean Spread with vegetable crudités.

Zucchini Soup
Reserve a portion for lunch tomorrow.

SERVES 4
21 oz. zucchinis, sliced
2 onions, chopped
3 cups water
1 tbsp fresh chives, chopped

1. Place the zucchinis, onion, and 2 tbsps of the water in a non-stick saucepan and cook over a gentle heat for 5–10 minutes to soften but not color.
2. Add the remaining water, bring to a boil, and simmer for 5 minutes.
3. Remove from heat, allow to cool slightly, and then blend in a food processor or blender.
4. Spoon into warm bowls, sprinkle with chives, and serve.

Butter Bean Spread
This is also good when used as a topping for baked vegetables.

1 can organic butter beans
1/2 small onion, chopped
1 garlic bulb, peeled and chopped
2 tbsps chopped fresh parsley
2 tbsps chopped fresh dill
1 tbsp tahini
2 tsps miso paste
1 small garlic clove, peeled and chopped

1. Place all the ingredients in a food processor and blend until smooth.
2. Serve with fresh vegetable crudités of your choice.

Day 12

BREAKFAST

1 cup of warm water
1 cup of nettle or dandelion tea
followed by vegetable juice.

Vegetable Juice
SERVES 1
6 carrots
1 stick of celery
1/2 beet
1 cucumber

Push all the ingredients through
a juicer and drink slowly.

MID-MORNING SNACK
One mango with a handful of raspberries.

LUNCH
Zucchini Soup from yesterday, followed by salad.

Quickest Quinoa Salad
SERVES 1
2 oz. quinoa grain
small bag of mixed salad leaves
enough of each of the following—to your
taste—to make a good-sized bowl of salad:
cucumber
beet, cooked
scallions, sliced
endive, sliced
snow peas
parsley, chopped
hazelnuts (optional)

1. Rinse the quinoa, then cook in boiling
water for 10 minutes until tender. Drain
in a sieve under cold running water.
2. Cut the cucumber into cubes, the beets
into wedges, and toss in a bowl with the
quinoa, scallions, endive, washed
and trimmed snow peas, and the parsley.
3. Serve on a bed of mixed salad leaves
and sprinkle with hazelnuts.

IF YOU WANT A FANCY OPTION
Place the scallions in a mixture of 1 tbsp
umeboshi vinegar and 1 1/2 tbsps brown rice
vinegar an hour before preparing your salad.
Mix in with the quinoa salad, and add 3 raw
radishes before serving.

   This option is not really necessary, but
I just want you to be thinking ahead about
what you can do with food for a day when you
might want to experiment. You could add
onion to pickle too if you want to get fancy.

MID-AFTERNOON SNACK
Handful of mixed seeds.

DINNER

Haddock with Braised Fennel
A simple fish dish as an alternative to
the fish burger when you are in a hurry.
It contains the spice star anise, which
is good for flu-fighting.

SERVES 4
4 3¹/₂-oz. skinless haddock fillets
2 fennel bulbs, finely sliced, core removed
2 star anise
1 cup cold water
1 lemon, sliced
1 tbsp black olives (optional)

1. Preheat the oven to 350°F.
2. Place the fennel in a baking dish or
roasting pan, add the star anise and water,
and bake for 15 minutes.
3. Remove the pan from the oven and lay the
fish on the fennel. Arrange the lemon slices
on the fish, then return it to the oven and
bake for 7–10 more minutes.
4. Remove the pan from the oven and allow
to stand for 5 minutes. Scatter with olives
and serve immediately.

**REMEMBER TO LEAVE YOUR BLACK BEANS
TO SOAK OVERNIGHT IN PLENTY OF WATER READY
FOR TOMORROW.**

Nothing beats the taste
of freshly blended
veggie juice. Freshly made
vegetable juices are a
potent source of nutrients,
and if you drink them on
a regular basis you'll enjoy
clearer skin, better energy
levels, and balanced
overall health.

Day 13

BREAKFAST

1 cup of warm water
1 cup of slippery elm tea
followed by a smoothie.

Strawberry and Peach Smoothie
SERVES 1
1 small basket strawberries
2 peaches, stoned and chopped
1 banana
1 pear, finely chopped

1. Blend the strawberries, peaches, and banana until smooth.
2. Pour over the chopped pear and serve.

MID-MORNING SNACK
Bowl of grapes.

LUNCH
Quinoa and Beet Salad.

Quinoa and Beet Salad
SERVES 2–3
3¹/₂ oz. quinoa grain, rinsed
3¹/₂ oz. green beans, trimmed and cut into 1" lengths
2¹/₂ oz. cucumber, halved lengthways and thinly sliced
2 vacuum-packed beets (no vinegar or sugar), drained and cut into thin wedges
1 scallion, trimmed and thinly sliced
¹/₂ small yellow pepper, de-seeded and thinly sliced
5 cherry tomatoes, halved
2 tbsps olive oil
2 tbsps freshly squeezed lemon juice
1 garlic clove, peeled and crushed
2 tbsps finely chopped fresh parsley

1. Cook the quinoa in a pan of boiling water for 12–15 minutes, or as instructed on the packet, until tender.
2. Cook the beans in a small pan of boiling water for 4 minutes until tender-crisp.
3. Drain the quinoa in a sieve under running water until cold. Press with the back of a spoon to remove the excess water. Tip into a serving bowl.
4. Drain the beans under running water until cold and add to the quinoa.
5. Add all the remaining ingredients and toss well together. Set aside for at least 15 minutes to allow the flavors to develop, then serve.

MID-AFTERNOON SNACK
Four baby radishes and a handful of Brazil nuts.

DINNER
Black Bean Soup with Avocado Drizzle and Wild Arugula.

Black Bean Soup with Avocado Drizzle and Wild Arugula

This Mexican-style soup is packed with flavor and makes a very satisfying supper dish. The black bean soup contrasts well in both color and taste with the avocado salsa.

SERVES 4

8 3/4 oz. **Black Beans, soaked overnight**
1 **onion, finely chopped**
2 **cloves garlic, peeled**
1 **leek, finely sliced**
2 **tbsps water**
1 **tsp olive oil**
1 **red pepper, finely chopped**
1 **qt. water or homemade stock**
1 **tsp coriander seeds, roughly ground**
2 **tbsps fresh parsley**
4 **tbsps fresh cilantro, finely chopped**
1 **ripe avocado, peeled, stoned, and finely chopped**
1/2 **red onion, finely chopped**
juice of 1 lime
1 3/4 oz. **arugula, roughly torn or chopped**

1. Soak the beans in cold water overnight. Drain and rinse well.
2. Place the onion, garlic, leek, water, and oil in a non-stick casserole dish, cover and cook over a low heat for 3–4 minutes until soft.
3. Add the water or stock, and the pepper. Bring to a boil and add the coriander seeds, parsley, fresh cilantro, and the beans. Simmer for 35–40 minutes.
4. Place the avocado and red onion in a small bowl with the lime juice and the arugula, stir gently to mix but not to mush the avocado.
5. Remove the soup from heat and allow to cool slightly. Transfer half the soup to the processor and process until smooth. Return the processed soup to the pan, stir to mix the two soups, and reheat gently.
6. Place a large spoonful of the avocado mixture in the center of four shallow bowls. Spoon the warmed soup around the avocado and serve immediately.

The Queen of Grains, quinoa is a fantastic source of protein, containing all the essential amino acids. Quinoa is your kidney supporter. And I consider your kidneys to be your bank account for life, so add interest with quinoa porridges, quinoa salads, and even my favorite, quinoa in soups.

Day 14

BREAKFAST

1 cup of warm water
1 cup of nettle tea
followed by fruit salad and a bowl
of Quick Oats.

Fruit Berry Salad
SERVES 1
1 small tub blueberries
1 small tub raspberries
1 small basket strawberries

Quick Oats

If you are still hungry, you can have
a bowl of oats, but you need to wait
20 minutes to let your fruit digest.

SERVES 1
3¹/₂ oz. oats
1²/₃ cups water or rice milk

1. Combine the oats with
the water or rice milk in a pan.
2. Bring to a boil, then lower the heat
and simmer for 15–20 minutes.
3. Season with a sprinkle of cinnamon.

MID-MORNING SNACK
Bowl of mung bean sprouts with a sprinkle of raw
shelled hemp, pumpkin, or sunflower seeds.

LUNCH
Black Bean Soup with Avocado Salsa from yesterday,
with some chopped raw endive leaves.

MID-AFTERNOON SNACK
Chop up a zucchini and top with hummus
and shredded carrot.

I want you to try every food
I put before you even if you
have never tried it before.
I need you to go beyond
your comfort zone of foods
that you usually eat. Also,
just because you don't love
something the first time
you try it does not mean
that you won't like it in the
future. Keep an open mind.

DINNER

Lemony Chicken Burgers served with a leafy green salad, or Tempeh Cutlets.

Lemony Chicken Burgers

Reserve two burgers for the following day. Allow them to cool, then cover and chill.

MAKES 6 BURGERS

2 tsps cold-pressed sunflower oil, plus extra for greasing
1³/₄ oz. onion, finely chopped
1 slim leek, trimmed and chopped
1 garlic clove, peeled and crushed
2 skinless, boneless free-range or organic chicken breasts (about 12¹/₂ oz.)
¹/₂ tsp organic wheat-free vegetable bouillon powder
1 tbsp freshly squeezed lemon juice
finely grated zest of a small lemon

1. Gently heat the oil in a pan with a little water and cook the onion, leek, and garlic over a low heat for 2 minutes until softened but not colored, stirring occasionally. Set aside to cool.
2. Preheat the oven to 390°F. Lightly oil a baking tray. Cut the chicken breasts into chunks and place in a food processor. Blend until fairly finely chopped but not mushy— you may have to remove the lid and push the chicken down once or twice until the right consistency is reached.
3. Transfer the chicken to a bowl and stir in the cooked onion, leek and garlic, bouillon powder, lemon juice, and zest. Mix well with clean hands and form into six balls.
4. Place the balls, evenly spaced apart, on the baking tray and flatten into burger shapes.
5. Bake for 10 minutes, then remove from the oven and turn over. Brush with a little more oil and return to the oven for 5 more minutes until cooked through.
6. Serve hot or cold with a large mixed salad.

VEGETARIAN ALTERNATIVE

Tempeh Cutlets

SERVES 4

8 oz. tempeh
large piece ginger, sliced into 9 pieces
4¹/₂ oz. watercress leaves
4¹/₂ oz. beansprouts
1³/₄ oz. daikon radish, cut into fine julienne
1 tsp sesame oil
3 tbsps water
dash of wheat-free tamari sauce

1. Arrange the ginger slices over the top of the tempeh.
2. Place the tempeh in a steamer basket over a pan of hot water, or in an electric steamer. Steam for 10 minutes.
3. Discard the ginger and slice the tempeh into ¹/₂" slices.
4. Arrange the watercress, beansprouts, and daikon on four serving plates.
5. Heat the sesame oil and water in a non-stick frying pan. Add the tempeh slices, cut side down, and water-fry for 1 minute. Turn the tempeh over and sprinkle with a little tamari sauce and cook for another minute.
6. Arrange the tempeh slices on the salad bed and spoon over a little of the cooking liquid. Serve immediately.

Day 15

BREAKFAST

1 cup of warm water
1 cup of sage herbal tea
followed by fruit salad.

Fruit Salad
SERVES 1
1 mango, stoned and chopped
1 banana
2 peaches, stoned and chopped
1/2 small tub blueberries
1/2 small tub raspberries

MID-MORNING SNACK
Juice of two apples and two pears.

Imagine what it's like to
feel absolutely fantastic.
That can easily be you.

LUNCH
Cashew Chicken Salad made with Chicken Burgers
from yesterday; or Cashew Tofu Salad.

Cashew Chicken or Cashew Tofu Salad
For the vegetarian alternative, substitute
tofu for the chicken. My salad is great for
packed lunches and can be prepared the
night before. Simply cool the vegetables
before adding the rest of the ingredients,
then cover and chill.

SERVES 2
1 tbsp olive oil
1 red pepper, cut into 1" pieces
2 1/2 oz. snow peas, trimmed
1 tsp wheat-free tamari sauce
2 cooked Lemony Chicken Burgers
    OR 2 1/2 oz. firm tofu cut into small squares
2 scallions, trimmed and sliced
1/4 oz. plain cashews, roughly chopped
1 romaine lettuce heart, leaves separated,
    washed, and drained
extra virgin olive oil and tamari sauce,
    to serve

1. Heat the oil in a large wok with a little
water. Sauté the pepper over a medium
heat for 2 minutes.
2. Add the snow peas and sauté for
30 seconds. Remove from the heat and
sprinkle with the tamari sauce.
3. Arrange the lettuce leaves in two bowls—
tearing in half first if the leaves are large.
Scatter the pepper and snow peas over
the lettuce.
4. Slice the chicken burgers and arrange
on top. Or if making tofu version, arrange
tofu squares on top. Sprinkle with the
scallions and nuts.
5. Drizzle with a little olive oil and extra
tamari sauce to serve.

MID-AFTERNOON SNACK

Veggie Juice or steamed corn on the cob spread with a little umeboshi plum sauce.

Veggie Juice
SERVES 1
6 carrots
2 celery stalks
4 sprigs parsley

DINNER

Gentle Lentil Curry with Tomato and Cilantro Relish.

Gentle Lentil Curry
Reserve a portion for lunch tomorrow.

SERVES 4
1 tbsp olive oil
1 medium onion, peeled and chopped
2 garlic cloves, peeled and crushed
1 tsp ground cumin
1/2 tsp ground turmeric
1/2 tsp ground ginger
5 1/4 oz. split red lentils, washed and drained
2 medium carrots, peeled and sliced
1 medium sweet potato, peeled and cut into 1" chunks
3 3/4 cups cold water
2 1/2 oz. green beans, trimmed and cut into 1" lengths
2 1/2 oz. frozen peas
sauerkraut (optional)
freshly cooked brown rice, to serve (optional)

1. Heat the oil in a large saucepan and cook the onion and garlic over a low heat for 3 minutes until softened but not colored.
2. Add the cumin, turmeric, and ginger and cook for 2 minutes, stirring regularly.
3. Stir in the lentils, carrots, and sweet potato. Turn in the oil for a few seconds, then add the cold water.
4. Bring to a boil and skim off any foam that rises to the surface. Boil for about 12–15 minutes until the lentils start to soften.
5. Add the beans and peas and continue to cook for 5 minutes more, stirring occasionally until the lentils are very soft and the vegetables are tender. Stir regularly, especially toward the end of the cooking time.
6. Serve with Tomato and Cilantro Relish, sauerkraut, and freshly cooked brown rice if desired.

Tomato and Cilantro Relish
SERVES 2
2 vine-ripened tomatoes, roughly chopped
2 scallions, trimmed and finely sliced
2 tbsps chopped fresh cilantro
1 tbsp freshly squeezed lime juice

Mix all the ingredients in a small bowl and leave for at least 30 minutes before serving.

Day 16

BREAKFAST

1 cup of warm water
1 cup dandelion tea
followed by a smoothie.

Soft Fruit Smoothie
SERVES 1
1 nectarine
1 soft pear
1 peach
1 tub berries

1. Blend until smooth.
2. You can always add a little pressed apple juice if this is too thick to blend.

MID-MORNING SNACK
Two celery stalks and half a cucumber, finely chopped. Serve with a dip if you fancy (see page 200).

LUNCH
Gentle Lentil Soup made with Gentle Lentil Curry from the day before.

Gentle Lentil Soup
SERVES 1
Reserved portion of Gentle Lentil Curry
1¼ cups water or stock

Simply put the curry and water in a food processor and blend until smooth. If you prefer a thicker or thinner soup add less or more water accordingly.

MID-AFTERNOON SNACK
Veggie Juice or one yellow pepper, sliced.

Veggie Juice
SERVES 1
6 carrots
1 cucumber
1 celery stalk
handful parsley
tiny piece of ginger

DINNER
Sushi Wraps.

Sushi Wraps

Wasabi paste (optional) can be purchased from Asian groceries and health food shops in small tubes. It adds a little extra to the avocado and chickpea paste, but it is not essential. Sushi daikon comes vacuum packed from the same sources, and once opened keeps well in the fridge. Reserve enough sushi for lunch the next day, wrapping the rolls in cling wrap and storing them in the fridge.

SERVES 2–3

3½ oz. short grain brown rice
1 tsp brown rice vinegar
1 avocado, peeled and stoned
7¾ oz. chickpeas drained
1" wasabi paste (optional)
   plus additional to serve
juice of half a lemon
¾ oz. toasted nori seaweed sheets (7 pieces)
3 sticks of celery, peeled and cut into
   fine strips
2 carrots, peeled and cut into fine strips
¾ oz. sushi daikon (or radish)
pickled ginger (or raw ginger)
wheat-free soy sauce

1. Place the rice in a small pan and cover with 1 cup water. Bring to a boil, cover, and simmer for 5 minutes.

2. Remove the pan from the heat and leave to stand for 15 minutes. Drain the rice in a colander.

3. Transfer the rice to a bowl, add the vinegar, and mix well.

4. Place the avocado, chickpeas, and wasabi (optional) in the food processor, process for 30 seconds, then add the lemon juice and process for a few more seconds.

5. Place a seaweed wrap on a clean working board. Spread a thin layer of the avocado mixture over the seaweed and cover with a layer of rice. Place a line of celery and carrot down the center of the rice.

6. Carefully roll up the sushi, and roll backward and forward a couple of times to tighten the roll. Place on a plate in the fridge and leave to chill for 5 minutes. Repeat the process with the remaining ingredients.

7. Slice the sushi rolls into 1" pieces. Serve with additional wasabi mustard, pickled ginger, and wheat-free soy sauce to taste.

Seaweeds are packed full of minerals, including calcium. I believe that low levels of dietary minerals are at epidemic levels in this country, so get into seaweeds to soak up more minerals.

Day 17

BREAKFAST

1 cup of warm water
1 cup nettle tea
followed by a smoothie.

Berry Delight
SERVES 1
1 small basket strawberries
2 soft pears
1 banana
1/2 cup water

Blend until smooth.

MID-MORNING SNACK
Bowl of grapes.

LUNCH
Sushi Wraps from yesterday, served with salad.

Oriental Style Salad
SERVES 1
1 zucchini
1/2 cucumber
1/2 red or yellow pepper
1 carrot
2 scallions, sliced
beansprouts
green salad leaves
FOR THE DRESSING
1 tbsp wheat-free tamari sauce
1 tsp sesame oil
2 tbsps water
1 clove garlic, crushed

1. Cut the zucchini, cucumber, peppers, and carrots into long thin sticks.
2. Toss with sliced scallions and rinsed beansprouts.
3. Mix together tamari sauce, sesame oil, water, and garlic.
4. Drizzle the dressing over the salad.
5. Serve over green salad leaves.

MID-AFTERNOON SNACK
One ripe avocado with a sprinkle of raw shelled hemp seeds and a teaspoon of hummus.

DINNER
Quick Cabbage and Bean Stew.

Quick Cabbage and Bean Stew
SERVES 2
1 onion, sliced
2 cloves garlic, crushed
3 carrots, peeled and sliced
1 sweet potato, peeled and diced
1 organic, wheat-free veggie stock cube
   or 1 tbsp miso paste
2^1/$_2$ pt. cold water
^{1}/$_2$ small savoy cabbage
14-oz. can navy beans
2 tbsps parsley, chopped

1. Place the onion, garlic, carrots, sweet potato, miso or stock, and 2^1/$_2$ pt. cold water in a pan. Bring to a boil.
2. Drain and rinse the navy beans.
3. Stir in the shredded cabbage, beans, and parsley.
4. Return to a boil and simmer until the cabbage is tender.

Eat cruciferous veggies as much as you can. Eat them raw and eat them cooked too. Vary the way you prepare them. Cabbage, broccoli, Brussels sprouts, turnip greens, watercress, and kale have been found to have potent cancer-fighting nutrients. They are also major helper foods for the liver and the processing of toxins, which is a must for any weight-loss quest.

Day 18

BREAKFAST

1 cup of warm water
1 cup of lemongrass tea
followed by a bowl of stewed prunes with
one ripe chopped pear, and a bowl of Oat
Groat Porridge.

Oat Groat Porridge
SERVES 1
4¹/₂ oz. oat groats
**1²/₃ cups rice milk or water—rice milk for
  extra sweetness**

1. Put the oat groats and water or rice milk
in a pot and bring to a boil. Lower the
heat and simmer until the groats thicken.
2. Turn off the heat and allow the porridge
to sit for a few minutes.
3. Sprinkle with cinnamon and serve.

MID-MORNING SNACK
One apple and one pear.

LUNCH
Miso soup (from packet) followed by vegetable crudités with Cashew and Brazil Nut Pâté.

Cashew and Brazil Nut Pâté
This mixture will keep well in the fridge
for up to two days.

SERVES 4
100g plain Brazil nuts, roughly chopped
100g plain cashews, roughly chopped
2 tsps olive oil
1 garlic clove, peeled and roughly chopped
1 tbsp freshly squeezed lemon juice
small bunch fresh parsley
4 tbsps cold water

1. Whiz all the ingredients together
in a food processor until almost smooth—
you may need to remove the lid and push
the mixture down a few times until the
right consistency is reached.
2. Serve with lots of fresh vegetable
crudités of your choice.

MID-AFTERNOON SNACK
Veggie Juice or four baby gem lettuce leaves with hummus, cherry tomatoes, grated carrot, and dill.

Veggie Juice
SERVES 1
3 broccoli florets
6 carrots
2 celery stalks
4 tomatoes

DINNER
Cinnamon Chicken with Minted Salad or Lentil
and Vegetable "Lasagna" with side salad.

Cinnamon Chicken with Minted Salad
SERVES 2

2 small boneless, skinless chicken breasts
   (total weight around 8 3/4 oz.)
1/2 tsp ground cinnamon
1/2 tsp ground cumin
2 tbsps chopped fresh cilantro
1 garlic clove, peeled and crushed
freshly squeezed juice of half a lemon
1 tsp virgin olive oil
lemon wedges, to serve

FOR THE SALAD

4 heaped tbsps frozen peas
2 scallions, trimmed
   and diagonally sliced
3 ripe vine tomatoes, roughly chopped
2 1/2 oz. cucumber, cut into 1/2" dice
2 tbsps roughly chopped fresh mint leaves
1 little gem lettuce, leaves separated,
   washed, and drained

1. Cut each chicken breast into eight
chunks and place in a non-metallic bowl.
Add the cinnamon, cumin, cilantro, garlic,
lemon juice, and olive oil. Cover and chill
for 30 minutes.

2. Preheat the oven to 390°F. Line a large
baking tray with non-stick foil.

3. Lift the chicken out of the marinade
using a fork and shake off any excess.
Place the pieces on the foil-lined tray,
spaced well apart.

4. Bake for around 15–18 minutes until
the chicken is cooked through.

5. Cook the peas in boiling water for
2 minutes. Drain in a sieve then plunge
into a bowl of cold water to cool.

6. Drain the peas once more and toss with
the scallions, tomatoes, cucumber,
and mint.

7. Divide the lettuce leaves between two
plates and top with the minted salad.

8. Serve the hot chicken with the salad
and lemon wedges for squeezing.

My mum used to tell me that I had to eat my oatmeal
because it would "stick tae my ribs and keep me warm."
What Mum did not know is that oats can do a lot more
than keep my insides warm. You can sow your wild oats,
literally. Oats have been found to increase sexual desire.

Lentil and Vegetable "Lasagna"

This recipe can be prepared ahead. Simply follow all the steps, then allow to cool. Cover and chill until required. It will keep for up to 24 hours. Cook from the fridge for 10–15 minutes until hot throughout.

SERVES 2
1 tbsp olive oil
1 medium onion, peeled and chopped
2 garlic cloves, peeled and crushed
1 yellow pepper, de-seeded and cut into
  1/2" dice
1 medium zucchini, trimmed and cut
  into 1/2" dice
2 1/2 oz. red split lentils, rinsed
14-oz. can chopped tomatoes
3 cups just-boiled water
2 tsps organic vegetable bouillon powder
1 large leek, trimmed to a length of 5 1/2"
1 oz. plain mixed nuts, chopped (optional)

1. Heat the oil in a large saucepan and gently water-fry the onion, garlic, pepper, and zucchini for 10 minutes until softened but not colored, stirring regularly.
2. Add the lentils and turn to coat in the oil.
3. Stir in the tomatoes, water, and bouillon powder. Bring to a boil, then reduce the heat slightly and simmer for about 25 minutes or until the lentils are tender and the liquid is reduced and thickened. Stir regularly, especially toward the end of the cooking time.

4. While the lentils are cooking, bring a large pan of water to a boil. Cut the leek in half lengthways and separate the layers. Add the leek to the boiling water and cook for 5 minutes or until very tender.
5. Preheat the oven to 390°F.
6. Drain the leek in a colander and cool under cold running water.
7. Remove the lentil mixture from the heat and spoon a third into the base of a 1 1/2 qt. rectangular ovenproof dish. Arrange half the sliced leek over the lentils. Top with another third of the lentils and the remaining leek. Finish with the rest of the lentil mixture and sprinkle with the nuts if using.
8. Bake for 15 minutes until hot.
9. Serve with a lightly dressed mixed salad.

Day 19

BREAKFAST

1 cup of warm water
followed by Avocado and Lime Shake.

Avocado and Lime Shake
SERVES 2
1 ripe avocado, halved and stoned
freshly squeezed juice of 1 lime
3 fresh dates, skinned and stoned (or figs)
2 cups cold water

1. Using a dessertspoon, scoop the avocado flesh into a food processor or liquidizer.
2. Add the lime juice, dates, and water.
3. Blend until smooth and serve in tall glasses.

MID-MORNING SNACK
Bowl of fresh pineapple chunks or one plum and one peach.

LUNCH
Hearty Miso Soup with brown rice and spinach, followed by vegetable crudités and cashew dip.

Hearty Miso Soup
Simply make up a bowl of miso soup from the packet and add some cooked brown rice and fresh, raw spinach leaves.

Creamy Cashew Dip
This recipe makes enough to serve four, so save some for snacking on with crudités tomorrow.

2 tbsps cashew butter
2 tbsps just-boiled water
few drops tamari sauce

1. Blend the cashew butter with 2 tsps of the just-boiled water in a small bowl until smooth.
2. Gradually add the remaining water, stirring well between each addition.
3. Season with a few drops of tamari sauce and stir until creamy.
4. Serve with vegetable crudités of your choice.

MID-AFTERNOON SNACK
Handful of unsalted mixed nuts or seeds.

DINNER
Herb Baked Cod with Oven Roasted Vegetables.

Tomato and Herb Baked Cod
Save some veggies for tomorrow's lunch.

SERVES 2
2 5-oz. fresh, skinless cod fillets
2 vine-ripened tomatoes, sliced
1 good pinch dried mixed herbs

1. Preheat the oven to 390°F/Gas 6. Place the fillets of cod onto two squares of foil—each roughly 1½" larger than the fish itself. Bring the sides up slightly to create a shallow foil bowl. Place on a baking tray.
2. Top each fillet with three slices of tomato and season with a pinch of dried herbs.
3. Bake for about 12 minutes until the fish is cooked—it should look opaque and flake easily.
4. Lift carefully onto two warmed plates, slide off the foil, and drizzle with the cooking juices to serve.

Simple Roasted Vegetables
SERVES 3–4
2 medium zucchinis, trimmed and cut into ½" slices
1 red pepper, de-seeded and cut into 1" pieces
1 yellow pepper, de-seeded and cut into 1" pieces
8 shallots, peeled and halved (quartered if large)
2 tbsps olive oil

1. Preheat the oven to 390°F.
2. Place the zucchinis, peppers, and shallots on a large baking tray. Drizzle with the oil and toss together lightly.
3. Bake for 35 minutes until tender and lightly browned, carefully turning halfway through the cooking time. Serve piping hot.

SOAK YOUR BARLEY OVERNIGHT TO READY FOR MAKING BREAKFAST SOUP.

If you want something sweet, opt for a piece of fruit or a root vegetable. They taste naturally sweet and should satisfy any sweet desires. And the more you chew your foods, the sweeter they taste.

Day 20

BREAKFAST

1 cup of warm water
1 cup of nettle tea
followed by melon slices and Breakfast
Barley Soup.
Remember to wait 20 minutes between
eating the fruit and the soup.

Breakfast Barley Soup
Soak the barley overnight, otherwise
you will have to call in late for work!
When you soak a grain like barley, it
makes the cooking more rapid.

SERVES 1
4 tbsps pearl barley
2 sachets white miso
4 shitake mushrooms

1. Drain the barley.
2. Bring ½ cup water to a boil
and add the barley.
3. Bring back to a boil, lower the
heat, and simmer for 10 minutes.
4. Add the white miso and shitake
mushrooms, simmer for five more
minutes, and then serve.

MID-MORNING SNACK
Two pears.

LUNCH
Oven Roasted Veggies from yesterday, with arugula
leaves and couscous.

Oven Roasted Veggies
SERVES 1
reserved portion of oven roasted vegetables
1 tbsp cider vinegar
2 tbsps pine nuts
a handful of arugula leaves
olive oil

1. Toss the oven roasted vegetables with
the cider vinegar, pine nuts, and arugula
leaves.
2. Drizzle with a little extra olive oil to serve.
3. Serve with a small bowl of plain couscous if
you feel extra hungry.

MID-AFTERNOON SNACK
Creamy Cashew Dip (see Day 19) with vegetable crudités.

DINNER
Bean Cassoulet with brown rice.

Bean Cassoulet
SERVES 2
1 onion, finely chopped
1 leek, washed and cut into $1/2$" pieces
2 cloves garlic
1 tsp olive oil
2 tbsps water
1 $10^{1}/_{2}$-oz. can no salt, no sugar
   flageolet beans, drained
1 7-oz. can no salt, no sugar
   borlotti beans, drained
2 sprigs of rosemary
1 tsp fennel seeds
few sprigs of thyme
1 tbsp millet flour
3 tomatoes, de-seeded and finely chopped
2 tbsps parsley

1. Place the onion, leek, garlic, oil, and water in a non-stick pan and cover and cook for 4–5 minutes until soft.
2. Transfer to an earthenware dish and mix in the beans. Scatter with the herbs (except parsley) and half the tomatoes.
3. Preheat the oven to 350°F.
4. Bake the cassoulet for 10 minutes. Remove from the oven and give the mixture a stir. Then sprinkle on the millet flour. Return to the oven and bake for 10 more minutes.
5. Sprinkle over the remaining tomatoes and parsley and serve with brown rice or a green salad.

When eating fruit, keep your melons separate from your other fruits. Melon digests faster than all other fruits. If you mix them with other fruits, you will be fermenting away in your gut and you know what that means ... GAS!

Day 21

BREAKFAST

1 cup of warm water
1 cup of sage tea
followed by a smoothie.

Berry, Mango, and Banana Smoothie

In the winter, you could always warm up the fruit for a change—but if you want to pour your warm smoothies over fruit, make sure the fruit is raw.

SERVES 1
1 tub raspberries
1 mango, stoned and chopped
1 banana

Blend until smooth.

MID-MORNING SNACK
Bowl of grapes.

LUNCH
Fennel, Cauliflower, and Celery Salad.

Fennel, Cauliflower, and Celery Salad

Fresh miso paste is available at the chilled counter at health food shops and is a good base for salad dressings as well as soups and stews.

SERVES 4
11 oz. fresh cauliflower florets
7 oz. celery, sliced
7 oz. fennel bulb, cored and chopped
4 tsps shelled hemp seeds
FOR THE DRESSING
2 tsps fresh miso paste with hemp
2 tbsps mirin
juice of 1 lemon

1. Steam the cauliflower florets for 3 minutes until just tender.
2. Mix in a bowl with the celery and fennel.
3. In a small jar, mix the miso paste, mirin, and lemon juice. Mix or shake well.
4. Pour the dressing over the salad, sprinkle with the seeds, and serve.

MID-AFTERNOON SNACK
Veggie Juice or a handful of salt-free organic almonds (if you can soak the almonds first in water they will be even easier to digest).

Veggie Juice
SERVES 1
1 cucumber
6 carrots
1 fennel
1/2 beet

DINNER
Speedy Sweet Potato Soup and Shitake Mushroom and Green Bean Salad with Sesame and Scallion Dressing.

Speedy Sweet Potato Soup

Save some for lunch tomorrow. If you don't have a stick blender, allow the soup to cool before blending in a food processor or liquidizer until smooth. Return to the pan and heat through gently.

SERVES 4
1 medium onion, peeled and roughly chopped
1 garlic clove, peeled and crushed
2 sweet potatoes, peeled and cut into
   1" chunks
2 medium carrots, peeled and thinly sliced
3¹/₃ cups just-boiled water
¹/₂ vegetable stock cube

1. Put all the ingredients in a saucepan and bring to a boil. Simmer for about 15 minutes until the vegetables are very tender.
2. Remove from the heat. Cool for a few minutes, then blend using a stick blender until smooth.
3. Add some extra water if necessary and warm through gently to serve.

Shitake Mushroom and Green Bean Salad with Sesame and Scallion Dressing

Furikake—a combination of black and white sesame seeds, nori seaweed, and red shiso leaves—is available from health food shops and Asian groceries. If you can't find it then use sesame seeds.

SERVES 2
2¹/₂ oz. green beans, ends trimmed
2 oz. mushrooms, preferably shitake, stalks removed and finely sliced
1 tbsp furikake seasoning
FOR THE DRESSING
2 scallions, white part only
1 tsp sesame oil
1 tbsp brown rice vinegar

1. Bring a small pan of water to a boil, add the beans, and cook for 1 minute. Drain and rinse well under cold running water.
2. In a small bowl mix the scallions, oil, and vinegar.
3. Arrange the beans on a serving plate and top with the sliced mushrooms. Spoon over the dressing then scatter with furikake and serve.

REMEMBER TO SOAK YOUR BLACK BEANS FOR TOMORROW—3 ¹/₂ OZ. IN PLENTY OF COLD WATER OVERNIGHT.

Day 22

BREAKFAST

1 cup of warm water
1 cup lemon balm tea
followed by a fruit salad of seasonal fruits,
and if you are still hungry, a bowl of oatmeal.
Pop a cup of chickpeas into water and soak
until tomorrow (this is for a snack).

Fruit Salad
Stewed apples and prunes served in
a warmed breakfast bowl, garnished
with a pinch of cinnamon.

Quick Oatmeal with Cinnamon and Vanilla
SERVES 1
3¹/₂ oz. oats
1²/₃ cups water
1" stick of cinnamon
vanilla pod, split in half lengthways

1. Place the oats and water in a small
saucepan and place over a moderate to high
heat, stir well, then add the cinnamon and
vanilla pod.
2. Bring to a boil without stirring. Simmer for
1 minute while stirring, until the mixture
becomes thick and creamy.
3. Remove from the heat when it reaches
your preferred consistency. Pour into a bowl
and discard the vanilla and cinnamon.
Serve immediately.

MID-MORNING SNACK
One tub of blueberries.

LUNCH
Speedy Sweet Potato Soup with salad.

Carrot and Pea Salad with Fresh Ginger
SERVES 1
4¹/₂ oz. carrot, peeled
2 oz. shelled fresh peas
freshly grated ginger, to taste
¹/₂ tbsp brown rice vinegar

1. Slice the carrot very finely, if possible
with a mandolin, and then place in a bowl
with the peas.
2. Grate some fresh ginger to taste,
add it to the peas and carrot.
3. Pour over the vinegar and serve.

MID-AFTERNOON SNACK
Handful of raw sugar snap peas or snow peas
and a handful of pumpkin seeds.

**Vegetable Rissoles with raw snow peas and
Sweet Corn Relish.**

Vegetable Rissoles

Use a good quality non-stick pan, and there is no need to use any more than a slight wipe of oil over the surface before cooking the rissoles.

SERVES 4
100g black beans
1/4 oz. arame seaweed
1 medium onion, finely chopped
1 tsp oil and 1 tbsp water
1/2 yellow pepper, finely diced
3 1/2 oz. peeled, grated swede
3 1/2 oz. zucchini, grated
2 tbsps chopped parsley
1 clove garlic, peeled and finely chopped
3 1/2 oz. millet flour
a little oil to grease

1. Soak the beans in a bowl of cold water overnight. Drain them and put them in a pan of cold water. Bring to a boil and simmer for 45 minutes. Drain and mash with a potato masher.
2. Soak the arame in cold water for 10 minutes and drain.
3. Place the onion in a non-stick pan with 1 tsp of oil and 1 tbsp of cold water, water fry gently to soften but do not brown.

4. Mix the cooked beans, arame, pepper, swede, zucchini, parsley, and garlic and stir well. Then mix in the millet flour.
5. Form into eight round balls.
6. Preheat a non-stick pan and take a little oil on a pastry brush and lightly oil the surface of the pan. Place four balls in the pan and with a flat spatula press down to flatten. Cook for 2–3 minutes until golden in color. Turn the rissoles over and cook for 2–3 more minutes until golden in color. Remove from the pan and repeat with the other rissoles.
7. Serve with raw snow peas, a squeeze of lemon juice, and Sweet Corn Relish.

Sweet Corn Relish

This will keep for 1–2 days in the fridge.

SERVES 4
5 1/4 oz. organic canned sweet corn
1/2 red pepper, finely diced
1/2 red onion, finely diced
2 tsps cider vinegar

Mix all the ingredients together and place in a clean jar until required.

Go for shitakes. These mushrooms have been found to have powerful, immune-enhancing properties. I want my clients to develop strong immune systems, so it's a good veggie to toss into salads, soups, and stews. Other interesting varieties are reishi, maitake, and enochi.

Day 23

BREAKFAST

1 cup of warm water
1 cup of dandelion tea
followed by a smoothie.

Peach, Apricot, and Banana Smoothie
SERVES 1
2 ripe peaches, halved and stoned
4 apricots
1 banana
¹/₂ cup water

Blend until smooth.

MID-MORNING SNACK
Bowl of sprouted mung beans sprinkled with
sesame seeds and a squeeze of lemon.

LUNCH
Avocado Stuffed with Black-Eyed Peas.

Avocado Stuffed with Black-Eyed Peas
Share this one with friends. They will
love this dish.

SERVES 2
1 avocado, halved, pit removed
squeeze of lemon juice
10¹/₂-oz. can of black-eyed peas, drained
   (You will only use half of the can here,
   save the rest for tomorrow)
3¹/₂ oz. cherry tomatoes, halved
1 scallion, chopped
¹/₂ tbsp cider vinegar
1 tbsp fresh basil

1. Place the avocado halves on serving
plates and sprinkle over the lemon juice.
2. Mix all the other ingredients together
and spoon into the avocados.
3. Serve immediately.

MID-AFTERNOON SNACK
Remember the chickpeas you soaked overnight?
They should now be just starting to sprout and so will
be packed with food enzymes. Drain and serve.

DINNER
Vegetable juice made from carrot, cucumber, and celery, followed by Asparagus Risotto.

Asparagus Risotto
Reserve a portion for tomorrow's lunch.

SERVES 4
1 bunch fresh asparagus
1 leek, halved and thinly sliced,
reserve the trimmings
1 qt. water
1 bay leaf
2 cloves garlic
1 tsp olive oil
2 tbsps water (for water frying)
10¹/₂ oz. short grain brown rice
2 tbsps flat leaf parsley
1 tbsp lemon juice
handful fresh arugula

1. Take the asparagus spears and snap the tough base from the stem. The asparagus will naturally break at the best point. Chop the asparagus into ¹/₂" pieces.
2. Place the leek trimmings and the discarded asparagus bases in a medium-sized pan, pour in the water, and bring to a boil. Add the bay leaf and leave to simmer.
3. In a non-stick frying pan heat the oil with 2 tbsps water and add the sliced leek and garlic. Cook for 5 minutes to soften but not color, then spoon in 2 tbsps of the asparagus water from the simmering pan.
4. Add the rice and cook for a few minutes stirring continuously. Then add 1 cup of the simmering asparagus water, cook for a few minutes until the rice absorbs all the water, and then add an additional cup of asparagus water.
5. Continue to add the hot asparagus liquid to the rice and cook over a gentle heat for approximately 30 minutes. The rice should require about 3¹/₃ cups of liquid. Discard the leek and asparagus trimmings.
6. Add the chopped asparagus to the rice, stir well, and simmer for 5 more minutes. Add the parsley and lemon juice. If required, add a little more stock. The rice should be tender and moist.
7. Serve the risotto in warmed soup plates and scatter with the fresh arugula.

If you want to lose weight, eat raw shelled hemp seeds. I call it my Weight Loss Seed. Raw shelled hemp contains the perfect ratio of the good fats that will help to burn fat in your body. It has a fabulous mineral profile and a good source of the much needed, sex-boosting nutrient zinc. Use raw shelled hemp seeds liberally as a snack, or in soups, stews, and dips.

Day 24

BREAKFAST

1 cup of warm water with a squeeze of lemon
1 cup of sage tea
followed by a Peach and Mango Smoothie.

Peach and Mango Smoothie
SERVES 1
1 mango, stoned and chopped
1 peach, stoned and chopped
1 banana, sliced
1/2 cup water
1 small tub blueberries

1. Blend all ingredients (except blueberries) until smooth.
2. Add more water if you want a thinner consistency.
3. Pour over the blueberries and drink.

MID-MORNING SNACK
Juice of a pink grapefruit and two apples or grapefruit segments.

LUNCH
Asparagus Risotto from yesterday, with Southern Style Black-Eyed Pea Salad.

Southern Style Black-Eyed Pea Salad with Red Onions and Peppers
Remember the black-eyed peas you had left over yesterday? Here's where you use them. This salad will keep well in the fridge for three days.

remainder of 10½-oz. can
    of black-eyed peas, drained
1/2 red onion, finely chopped
1/2 red pepper, cored, de-seeded,
    and finely chopped
1/2 yellow pepper, cored, de-seeded
    and finely chopped
FOR THE DRESSING
1 tbsp fresh cilantro, chopped
1/2 tsp Dijon mustard
1/2 tbsp cider vinegar
1/2 tbsp olive oil

1. Mix the beans, onion and peppers together.
2. Place the dressing ingredients in a jar and shake well.
3. Pour the dressing over the beans, stir well, cover, and chill.
4. Leave to marinade for 2–3 hours before serving for extra flavor, or simply eat straightaway.

MID-AFTERNOON SNACK
Veggie Juice or a red or yellow pepper, sliced.

Veggie Juice
SERVES 1
1 fennel
1/2 beet
4 celery stalks

DINNER
Salmon and Savoy Cabbage "Lasagna."

Salmon and Savoy Cabbage "Lasagna"
This dish gets its name from the layers
of cabbage and salmon that resemble
a traditional lasagna. It is full of flavor
and is really good for entertaining.

SERVES 4
1 large savoy cabbage
2 tsps sesame oil
3 tbsps boiling water
zest of 1 lemon
2 tsps brown rice vinegar
1 tsp wheat-free soy sauce
10 oz. fillet of salmon
8 scallions, finely chopped

1. Remove the outer leaves from the cabbage
and discard. Take 5 leaves from the cabbage
and remove the tough central vein. This will
leave a small "V" shape in the leaf.
2. Bring a large pan of water to a boil and add
the 5 leaves. Boil for 2 minutes. Drain
and refresh in cold water.
3. Finely shred the remaining cabbage and
place in a non-stick pan with the sesame oil
and boiling water. Place on a moderate heat
and cook until the cabbage has just wilted,
than add the lemon zest, rice vinegar, and
soy sauce. Remove from the heat and leave
in the pan to cool.

4. Place the salmon fillet on a chopping
board and with a sharp knife slice the fish
horizontally into ¹/₈" slices.
5. Take a large piece of greaseproof paper
and place a cabbage leaf in the center. Cover
with half of the salmon slices. With a slotted
spoon, place half of the shredded cabbage
mixture on top. Cover with a second cabbage
leaf and repeat the process until you have
completed the lasagna.
6. Drizzle a little of the cooking juice from
the shredded cabbage over the top. Wrap the
paper firmly around the salmon and cabbage.
7. Place the parcel in a bamboo steamer
over a pan of boiling water and steam for
7–10 minutes. The parcel will feel firm to
the touch.
8. Remove from the steamer, unwrap, and
slice into four wedges. Transfer to 4 warm
serving plates and drizzle over any remaining
juices.
9. Scatter the chopped scallions over
the top and serve immediately.

Day 25

BREAKFAST

1 cup of warm water
1 cup of nettle and dandelion tea combined
followed by Quinoa Vanilla Porridge.

Quinoa Vanilla Porridge
SERVES 2
5¼ oz. quinoa grains
½ vanilla pod
1½ cups water or rice milk

1. Combine the quinoa, vanilla pod, and
water or rice milk in a pan.
2. Bring to a boil, then lower the heat
and simmer for approximately 10 minutes, or
until the grains are translucent.
3. Take off the heat and allow to stand
for a few minutes before serving.

MID-MORNING SNACK
Two fresh figs, or dried (unsulphured) if you can't get fresh.

LUNCH
Watercress Soup with Turnip, and Avocado, Tomato, and Basil Salad.

Watercress Soup with Turnip

This soup has a fantastic peppery taste and is best made whilst organic watercress is in season through the summer months. It should be made when the watercress is very fresh, and cooked and eaten on the same day to preserve its nutritional value. If watercress is unavailable, then replace with lettuce leaves.

SERVES 2
1 bunch (4½ oz.) watercress (or lettuce)
1 onion, finely chopped
1 tsp olive oil
2 tbsps water
3½ oz. white turnips, peeled and chopped
3 cups homemade stock or water

1. Trim the leaves from ½ bunch of the watercress (if using) and set aside for garnish.
2. Place the onion, oil, and water in a medium-sized pan, cover, and cook until soft but not colored.
3. Add the turnips and stock, bring to a boil and simmer for 20–30 minutes until the turnips are soft when pierced with a knife.
4. Add the watercress (or lettuce) and cook for barely 1 minute, remove from the heat, and allow to cool slightly.
5. Pour the soup into the processor or blender and blend until smooth.
6. Serve in four warmed serving bowls and garnish with the reserved watercress leaves.

Avocado, Tomato, and Basil Salad
SERVES 2
2 ripe avocados, halved
4 medium vine-ripened tomatoes, sliced
2 handfuls fresh basil leaves
½ oz. pine nuts
2 tbsps extra virgin olive oil
1 tsp good quality balsamic vinegar

1. Stone the avocados and slice thickly. Peel off the skin and discard.
2. Arrange the avocado slices on two serving plates and top with the tomatoes and basil leaves. Sprinkle with the pine nuts.
3. Drizzle with olive oil and balsamic vinegar to serve.

MID-AFTERNOON SNACK
Tub of blueberries or raspberries.

DINNER
Chinese Cabbage Casserole.

Chinese Cabbage Casserole
Reserve a portion for lunch tomorrow.

SERVES 4
1 qt. water
1" piece fresh ginger, sliced
1 tsp coriander seeds, crushed
1 clove garlic, peeled
21 oz. Chinese cabbage
3½ oz. daikon (or radish), peeled
   and cut into julienne or matchsticks
3½ oz. carrots, peeled and sliced
4 tbsps fresh cilantro, chopped
1 tsp sesame oil
1 tsp wheat-free soy sauce
1 tbsp sesame seeds
¾ oz. arame soaked in cold water
   for 10 minutes and drained

1. Place the water, ginger, coriander seeds, and garlic in a medium to large saucepan. Bring to a boil.
2. Add the cabbage, daikon, and carrots and simmer for 5 minutes.
3. Remove from the heat and stir in half the cilantro.
4. Spoon into soup bowls and drizzle over the oil, soy sauce, sesame seeds, remaining cilantro, and arame. Serve.

SOAK 2¾ OZ. ADZUKI BEANS IN PLENTY OF COLD WATER OVERNIGHT TO READY FOR TOMORROW.

Day 26

BREAKFAST

1 cup of warm water
1 cup of spearmint or fennel tea
followed by a smoothie.

Strawberry Smoothie
SERVES 1
1 small punnet strawberries, hulled
1/2 tub raspberries
2 ripe pears, cored and chopped
1 apple, peeled and chopped
1 cup water

Blend all the ingredients until smooth.

MID-MORNING SNACK
Hummus with a selection of seeds:
pumpkin, sunflower, or raw shelled hemp.

LUNCH
Chinese Cabbage Casserole from yesterday, served with
a steamed corn on the cob that you have rubbed with
umeboshi plum sauce.

MID-AFTERNOON SNACK
Half a cucumber, finely chopped.

DINNER
Adzuki Bean Mini Burgers with Onion Gravy.

Reserve a portion of Burgers
and Onion Gravy for tomorrow.

Always, always opt for brown rice over white if you
want to have energy and stay slim. White rice is
stripped of too many nutrients and tends to behave
like sugar in the body. Brown rice is a good source of
B vitamins that are critical for adrenal function and
weight balance. Recent research has found that eating
a diet rich in whole grains such as brown rice can
help to control weight gain. So now you know…

Adzuki Bean Mini Burgers

If you boil the soaked adzuki beans for
about 40 minutes until very soft, they
will blend better in the food processor.

MAKES 12 BURGERS

2¹/₂ oz. mixed unsalted nuts, roughly
   chopped (I use pine nuts)
6¹/₄ oz. soft cooked adzuki beans
2 tbsps tahini (sesame paste)
1³/₄ oz. roughly chopped onion
2 tbsps chopped fresh parsley
1 tsp organic vegetable bouillon powder
1 tsp olive oil

1. Preheat the oven to 390°F.
Cover a baking tray with non-stick foil.
2. Place the nuts in a food processor and
blend until finely ground. Add the adzuki
beans, tahini, onion, parsley, and stock.
3. Blend until the mixture forms an almost
smooth, thick paste—you may have to remove
the lid and push the mixture down once or
twice until the right consistency is reached.
Roll into twelve small balls with clean hands
and place on the baking tray. Flatten into
small burger shapes.
4. Brush the burgers lightly with the oil
and bake for 10 minutes. Remove from the
oven and carefully turn over using a spatula.
Return to the oven for 5–7 more minutes until
the burgers are cooked through and lightly
browned.
5. Serve the burgers with Onion Gravy or
Zesty Avocado Mayo (page 98), plus a large
mixed salad or lots of seasonal vegetables.

Onion Gravy

3 onions
3 tbsps olive oil
2 tsps tamari sauce

1. Sweat the onions in the olive oil on
a low heat for 15 minutes until soft and
translucent. You are not frying them.
2. Add a little water under the onions and
cook them for another 10–15 minutes.
3. Blend the onions and pour into a bowl.
Add the tamari sauce and serve.

Day 27

BREAKFAST

1 cup of warm water
1 cup of nettle tea

Fruit Smoothie
It's got to be a smoothie and one that
you concoct. So get busy. And let me
know what you come up with.

MID-MORNING SNACK
One tub of blueberries.

LUNCH
Leftover Adzuki Bean Burgers with Onion Gravy
from yesterday.

MID-AFTERNOON SNACK
Bowl of raw sauerkraut (rinsed).

DINNER
Minced Turkey Meatballs with Surprise Tomato Sauce
and crunchy salad, or Chickpea Vegetable Stew.

**Minced Turkey Meatballs with
Surprise Tomato Sauce**
The sauce is optional and the meatballs
are equally delicious simply served with
a leafy green salad and a squeeze of lemon.

SERVES 4
18 oz. fresh turkey mince, preferably
   organic or free-range
1 medium onion, peeled and finely chopped
1 garlic clove, peeled and crushed
1 small bunch fresh cilantro, finely chopped
$1/2$ tsp organic wheat-free vegetable bouillon
   powder
FOR THE SAUCE
14-oz. can chopped tomatoes
1 garlic clove, peeled and chopped
1 medium onion, peeled and roughly chopped
1 celery stick, trimmed and thinly sliced
1 large carrot, peeled and thinly sliced
1 sweet potato, peeled and cubed
1 leek, trimmed and finely sliced
1 zucchini, trimmed and cubed
1 bay leaf (optional)

1. Place all the sauce ingredients in a large saucepan. Fill the empty tomato can with cold water and pour over the vegetables. Bring to a boil, then reduce the heat and simmer gently for 25–30 minutes until the vegetables are tender and the sauce is thick, stirring regularly.

2. Meanwhile, preheat the oven to 390°F. Place the turkey mince in a large bowl and, using clean hands, mix thoroughly with the onion, garlic, cilantro, and bouillon powder.

3. Form the mince mixture into twenty small balls and place on a baking tray lined with foil. Bake for 12–15 minutes, turning halfway through the cooking time, until the turkey is lightly browned and cooked through.

4. Allow the cooked sauce to cool for 5 minutes. Discard the bay leaf, if using, and then carefully blend the sauce until smooth.

5. Return to the pan and stir in the meatballs. Heat through gently together until the sauce is hot.

6. Serve with a crisp, crunchy raw salad.

Chickpea Vegetable Stew

SERVES 2

1 red onion, sliced
2 garlic cloves, crushed
1 tbsp hemp oil or olive oil
1 red pepper, diced
1 zucchini, sliced
1 leek, sliced
1 14-oz. can of no salt, no sugar chickpeas
1.2 cups cold water
**2 tsps wheat-free vegetable bouillon
    stock powder**
handful baby spinach leaves

1. Sweat the onion and garlic in the oil over a low heat until the onion is soft.

2. Stir in the red pepper, zucchini, and leek. Rinse the chickpeas and add them to the onion and pepper mixture.

3. Add the water and bouillon powder and bring to a boil. Reduce the heat and simmer for 6–8 minutes until the vegetables are just tender.

4. Stir in the baby spinach leaves at the last moment and serve with freshly cooked brown rice.

Day 28

BREAKFAST

1 cup of warm water
1 cup of nettle tea
followed by Warm Fruit.

Warm Fruit
1 apple
1 pear
2 peaches
2 apricots

Chop all the fruit and warm through in
a pan with 1/2 cup of pressed apple juice
before serving.

MID-MORNING SNACK
Two grated carrots and one grated beet with a handful
of alfalfa sprouts and a squeeze of lemon.

LUNCH

Chilled Fennel Soup with Avocado and Cucumber

SERVES 2
1 tsp olive oil
2 fennel bulbs, chopped, with the tough
    core removed
1/2 daikon (or radish), peeled and chopped
1 bay leaf
1 tsp coriander seeds
1 cup vegetable stock
1/2 cucumber, finely diced
1 avocado, finely diced
juice of 1/2 lemon

1. Heat the oil in a non-stick pan, add a little
water, and sweat the fennel for 2 minutes.
2. Add the daikon, bay leaf, coriander seeds,
and vegetable stock and simmer until the
fennel is tender (about 20–25 minutes).
3. Pass the mixture through a Mouli
or coarse sieve. Allow to cool.
4. Mix the cucumber with the avocado and
the lemon juice. I think it tastes great when
it is all blended together. You can also simply
stir into the soup. Either way, chill before
serving.

Do not eat standing up or when running
around on the go. Sit down when you are
eating a meal or a snack. You will digest
your food far more effectively when you
are relaxed.

Broccoli Salad with Pine Nuts

SERVES 2

1 head broccoli, cut into florets
1/2 red onion, diced
10 cherry tomatoes, halved
2 tbsps basil, chopped
2 tbsps pine nuts, lightly toasted
1 tbsp tamarind
juice of half a lemon

1. Bring a pan of water to a boil and blanch the broccoli for 1 minute.
2. Strain in a colander and run under cold water. Allow to drain. This prevents the broccoli from losing its color and nutrients.
3. Place the broccoli in a salad bowl with the onion, tomato, and basil.
4. Mix the pine nuts with the tamarind and lemon juice and spoon over the salad.

MID-AFTERNOON SNACK
Cucumber and carrot crudités with hummus, sprinkled with dill.

DINNER
Bean Sausages with Onion Gravy and freshly cooked vegetables.

Bean Sausages with Onion Gravy

If you are making this dish to serve 3, make 6 fat sausages instead of 8 thinner ones and cook for 1–2 minutes longer.

SERVES 3–4

3^1/$_2$ oz. shelled mixed nuts such as Brazil, hazelnut, almonds, walnuts, and pecans, roughly chopped
1^3/$_4$ oz. onion, roughly chopped
1 clove garlic, peeled and halved
10^1/$_2$-oz. can red kidney beans, drained and rinsed under cold water in a colander
2 tbsps roughly chopped fresh parsley
1 tsp organic vegetable bouillon powder
1 tsp virgin olive oil

FOR THE ONION GRAVY

1 tsp virgin olive oil
1^3/$_4$ oz. onion, thinly sliced
^{3}/$_4$ cup just-boiled water
2 tsps organic wheat-free tamari sauce
1^1/$_2$–2 tsps ground arrowroot blended with 2–3 tsps cold water

1. Preheat the oven to 390°F. Line a baking sheet with non-stick foil.
2. Place the nuts in a food processor and blend until very finely chopped.
3. Add the onion, garlic, kidney beans, parsley, and bouillon powder. Blend until the mixture forms an almost smooth, thick paste—you may have to push the mixture down with a spatula once or twice until the right consistency is reached.
4. Form the mixture into eight balls with clean hands, then roll into sausage shapes (about 3^1/$_2$" long) and place on the baking tray.
5. Brush the sausages all over with a little oil and bake for 10 minutes. Carefully remove the tray from the oven and turn the sausages over. Cook for a further 5–7 minutes until lightly browned and hot throughout.
6. While the sausages are cooking, prepare the gravy. Place the oil and onion in a small saucepan with 1 tbsp cold water and cook over a low heat for about 5 minutes until the onion is softened and very lightly browned, stirring regularly.
7. Add the just-boiled water and tamari sauce and bring to the boil. Stir in the arrowroot mixture—less arrowroot will make a thinner gravy—and cook for 1 minute, stirring constantly until the sauce is thickened and glossy.
8. Serve the sausages with the gravy and lots of freshly cooked vegetables.

Make green your favorite color and keep thinking green when it comes to mealtimes. So eat plenty of fresh, leafy greens, kale, collards, turnip greens, mustard greens, parsley, and bok choy. Greens are packed with minerals, and we need lots of minerals to function at a top level.

level three

the Dr. Gillian detox

We hear about detox a lot. My message to you is that opting for a healthy lifestyle is more important than crash detoxing. Once you've followed my plan and are in the groove, then a cleansing detox can be great once every few months. In this chapter I'll give you a really simple two-day detox you can try when you feel like it.

Don't use detoxing as a substitute for a healthy diet.

A dear friend of mine from New York is the ultimate detox junkie. Barbara is often overweight and loves to gorge on hard cheeses—breakfast, lunch, and dinner—sometimes eating very large slabs at one sitting. She tells me that when no one is around she devours cakes, ice cream, and anything that sounds, looks, or smells like a potato chip. She loves living in New York City because she says it is the one place where she can call in for take-out at any time of the day or night, or even pop out in the early hours to get a large of tub of cookies-and-cream ice cream that she has been known to wolf down at four in the morning.

When I confront Barbara about her eating habits, she tells me not to worry. She says that she actually is very health-conscious because she detoxes on a regular basis at a center in California. During these intervals, she eats nothing but bean sprouts and drinks gallons of cucumber juice. But I have since learned that she is not as much of a goody-two-shoes as she would like us all to think. The last time I tried to contact her when she was at the center in California, she had disappeared. No one knew where she was. It turned out she had escaped in search of cherry pie and the next day had to order a colonic in the vain hope that she would redress the balance.

Barbara mistakenly believes that she can abuse her body at home, day in and day out, and then counteract the impact every few months with a severe detox. But it just doesn't work that way. Detoxes are fine, but not at the expense of a daily, healthy eating plan. But as part of a healthy lifestyle they are a fantastic way to cleanse and replenish.

As part of a healthy lifestyle,
detoxes are a fantastic way
to cleanse and replenish.

WHY DETOX AT ALL?

The body is naturally detoxing every day. However, depending on what you eat, how you live your life, where you live, and how your body performs, natural detoxing often needs some help.

The colon is the body's sewage system. If the sewage system stops flowing efficiently, toxins collect in the colon and become a breeding ground for unhealthy bacteria. Blood capillaries lining the colon wall begin to absorb toxins into the bloodstream, and this lowers the overall performance of bodily functions. Over time, these toxins can build up in the body, settling in the various organs and causing fatigue, digestive problems, weight gain, and a variety of skin, hair, and health problems.

TOP DETOX FOODS

Artichokes	Fruit smoothies	Radishes
Asparagus	Garlic	Raw cabbage
Broccoli	Grapefruit	Raw food
Cauliflower	Green leaves	Sprouted seeds
Daikon	Hemp seeds (raw shelled)	Tarragon
Dandelion tea	Lemons	Turmeric
Endive	Lovage	Veggie juices
Fennel	Mung beans	Warm water
Flaxseeds	Nettle tea	Watermelon
Fruit salad	Papaya	

GETTING STARTED

Weekends are usually easier for a two-day detox. However, it is not set in stone that it must be done over a weekend. Just make sure that the detox is carried out over two consecutive days.

YOUR DETOX KIT

1 Foods and teas for the cleansing
2 Juicer or a shop nearby that can make juices for you
3 Blender
4 Skin brush
5 Two candles
6 Essential oils of myrrh and frankincense
7 A notepad
8 Lots of still bottled water if you do not have a filter (drink about 2 liters of water each day of the detox)
9 Flaxseeds
10 Hemp oil or extra virgin olive oil
11 Hot water bottle
12 Fun music to dance to
13 Fresh mint
14 A cup of castor oil
15 Cotton sheeting
16 Powdered acidophilus

Early to Bed, Early to Rise

I want you in your bed early for a week before your detox and during the detox. No later than 10:30 p.m. Sleep is an essential part of the process.

Deep Breathing

Upon waking up the day before your detox and during the two-day detox, sit on a hard-surfaced chair with your bare feet firmly planted on the floor.

► Feel the soles of your feet touching the surface of the floor
► Feel the area under your belly button with the palm of your hand
► Place the palm of your hand flat on that area
► Close your eyes and relax
► Breathe deeply, then as you breathe out say: *"I am healthy. I eat good food every day."*
► Repeat this affirmation 10 times

Bath Time

Take only short baths during the detox weekend. If you feel like having a hot bath, make sure that it is a 20-minute bath at most.

The night before your detox, soak two tablespoons of organic flaxseeds in a large bowl of hot water.

Stay at home or close to home on your detox days.

Day 1

UPON WAKING

Deep Breathing Exercise
(See page 165)

One Cup of Warm Lemon and Lime Water
A cup of warm water is a cleansing way
to start the day. Add a few squeezes of lemon
and a couple of squeezes of lime for even
greater effect. Take your time to drink it.
There is no need to rush.

One small cup of dandelion tea

Strain the flaxseeds that you have soaked
overnight and drink only the broth.

Exercise
Twenty-minute brisk walk.

Dry Skin Brush
Dry skin brushing speeds up the rate
at which toxins are expelled from the
body, because it stimulates blood cells
and lymph tissue, two key physiological
detoxification avenues.

Brush smoothly the soles of the feet,
working your way up the legs, then up
the arms and down the back. Brush in long,
sweeping movements toward your heart,
as it increases circulation and improves skin
tone and texture. Always brush lightly and
gently and avoid areas of broken skin,
thread veins, and varicose veins.

Take your shower after skin brushing.

BREAKFAST

Large Fruit Salad Berry Compote
¹/₂ **small tub blueberries**
¹/₂ **small tub raspberries**
¹/₂ **small basket strawberries**
Or more if you want

Berries are superb for the liver. Nourishing
the liver is key for detoxification.

1 mug of dandelion tea

MID-MORNING
Turn on your favorite piece of music, dance, and have fun.

Fruit Juice
¹/₂ **pineapple or more (simply pass
through the juicer and serve).**

Exercise
Before lunch, go for a brisk walk.

LUNCH

Warm Detox Broth

You are going to simmer these vegetables and drink only the broth. Please try to get organic vegetables whenever possible. Do not peel the veggies if they are organic.

6 carrots
3 large white potatoes
1 daikon or 4 radishes
2 turnips
1 cup parsley
4 celery stalks
1 garlic clove
1 strip of kombu (seaweed)

1. Fill a saucepan with 2½ qt. of water. Pop your veggies into the pot and bring to a boil.
2. Reduce the heat, put a lid on the pot, and simmer for 2 hours on a very low heat.
3. Strain the vegetables and drink a third of the broth. Save the rest for the evening and for tomorrow.

Detox Sprout Salad
SERVES 1
3½ oz. organic mung bean sprouts
1½ oz. celery, finely sliced
½ oz. Chinese cabbage, shredded
squeeze of lemon juice
6 endive leaves

1. Place the sprouts, celery, and cabbage in a salad bowl and mix well. Squeeze over the lemon juice.
2. Arrange the endive leaves on a plate, spoon over the mung bean sprout salad, and serve.

MID-AFTERNOON
Turn on your favorite piece of music and dance like crazy.

Vegetable Juice
6 carrots
1 cucumber
2 celery stalks
½ onion
handful of cabbage leaves

1 cup nettle tea

LATE AFTERNOON

Vegetable Juice
1 fennel
1 whole cucumber
2 celery sticks
(add a small piece of ginger if you feel cold and want to warm up)

1 cup of nettle tea

Exercise
Before dinner, go for a brisk walk.

DINNER
Eat early, around 6:00 p.m.

Detox Broth (see page 167)
Raw Pâté with Sprouts

Fresh Mint Tea
Take a generous handful of fresh mint leaves and steep in boiling water for a few minutes before drinking.

Raw Pâté
SERVES 2
2 tbsps torn fresh basil
1 tbsp chopped cilantro
7 oz. whole almonds, soaked
2¹/₂ oz. pine nuts
2 tbsps lemon juice
1 garlic clove

1. Place all ingredients in a food processor and blend until smooth.
2. Place in a small bowl and refrigerate.
3. Serve with mixed sprouts.

Dry skin brush and a short bath

Apply castor oil pack
Using a castor oil pack seems to increase detoxification through the liver and trigger the organs of elimination to open and release. It may also stimulate the lymphatics and improve circulation and the removal of toxins generally.

Find a piece of cotton fabric that, when folded so that it is four layers thick, will cover your abdomen from your hips to your chest. You can tear up an old cotton sheet for this. Fold the fabric into four layers and pour castor oil liberally onto the top layer of the fabric—about a cup of oil. Lie down and place the castor oil pack over your abdomen with the oiled layer of fabric against the skin. Cover it with a towel or some plastic wrap, for instance cling wrap, to prevent the oil reaching any linen or clothing.

Apply a hot water bottle to the liver and abdominal area. Hold in place for a minimum of an hour. If the hot water bottle cools, refill with hot water. You need to keep it as hot as possible for maximum benefits.

NOTE: PACKING WOULD NOT BE ADVISED DURING MENSTRUATION, PREGNANCY, OR LACTATION.

Meditation by candlelight

Place a white candle in a safe place so that it is about a foot in front of you. Make sure you can look at it without slouching or feeling uncomfortable. Sitting at a table is often the best position for this meditation.

Light the candle. Close your eyes and focus on your body and your center. Ground yourself in the moment by being aware of the ground, floor, chair, or whatever you are sitting on.

Open your eyes and look at the flame and pay attention to it—the colors, the movement, and the still place in the center of it.

You'll have thoughts. Let them go without worrying about them and bring your attention back to the candle. Do this for about 10 minutes.

The candle symbolically represents the burning away of any negative energies you may have attracted or created.

DAY TWO PREP

Soak 2 tbsps of organic flaxseeds in a large bowl of hot water.

For inspiration and motivation during the two-day detox, always remind yourself why you are embarking upon this cleansing program. It's a chance for you to purge toxic residues, and take care of your body, glands, organs, cells and general health.

BEFORE BED

Drink a cup of warm water an hour before bed. Just before bed, retrieve your notepad and take time to write down your thoughts about today. How do you feel? What emotions do you have? Don't hold back. Write down everything that comes into your head.

Keep your notepad and pen by your bed. If you have any dreams tonight, write them down upon waking.

10:00 p.m. BEDTIME

Day 2

You are going to drink loads of juice during Day 2. I don't want you just to drink one or two juices; I want you to drink lots of them to satisfy and cleanse your bowels, organs, and cells. This is not about depriving yourself. If you feel, "I want food, I'm hungry," then please drink more juice. You should be able to satisfy your hunger cravings, if you have any, by simply drinking enough juice.

A full day of drinking just fresh juice is one of the most efficient ways to dislodge mucus and catarrh, cleanse the organs—especially the kidneys, liver, and bowels—while simultaneously infusing nutrients and live enzymes into your body with the least amount of effort from your digestive system.

Obviously, if hunger and a dissatisfied feeling become overwhelming, then by all means please eat some solid vegetables or brown rice. It is not a problem if that's what you need to do the first time around.

You can consume one fruit smoothie and one fruit juice in the morning up until about 11:00 a.m. After that swap to veggie juices. You might also buy some powdered acidophilus from a health store and drink it with water toward the end of the day. The acidophilus will help to spur the growth of healthy bacteria.

A Word about the Juices

I want you to feel free to choose those vegetable juices that are right for you. If you find the taste of vegetable juices "hard going," then simply add some carrot juice (or apple) to the vegetable juice. Because carrots are a sweet-tasting vegetable, they will soften the taste of any other more sour vegetable. Celery and cucumber juices tend to have more neutral flavors too.

I have included times in the second day. If possible do try to stick to these—as you'll see you've got a lot of juicing to get through!

7:00 a.m. UPON WAKING

Deep Breathing Exercise (see page 165)

1 cup of warm water with a squeeze of lemon and lime
1/2 cup nettle tea mixed with 1/2 cup slippery elm tea

Exercise
Go for a 20-minute brisk walk.

8:00 a.m. BREAKFAST

Strain the flaxseeds you have been soaking overnight from the water and drink only the liquid.

Fruit Smoothie
4 peaches
2 pears
6 apricots
OR a nice big slice of watermelon if in season.

10:15 a.m. Vegetable Juice
handful alfalfa sprouts
4 celery stalks
1 cucumber
3 broccoli florets
1 garlic bulb

11:15 a.m. Dandelion tea

11:30 a.m. Go for a 20-minute brisk walk

NOON

Juicy Detox Smoothie
6 carrots
1 celery
1 ripe avocado
1 apple
squeeze of lemon
8 basil leaves

1. Juice the apple, celery, and carrots through your juicer.
2. Place the juice in your blender with the avocado and basil leaves.
3. Squeeze a dash of lemon into the blend and serve.

2:15 p.m. Vitality Juice
6 tomatoes
6 carrots
6 celery stalks
1 red pepper
1/2 beet
1 cucumber
1/4 onion
1/4 green cabbage head
6 green beans

4:00 p.m. Vegetable Juice (see Day 1)

5:00 p.m. Go for a 20-minute brisk walk

6:00 p.m. Detox Broth (see Day 1)

Detox Sprout Salad
SERVES 1
4¹/₂ oz. cucumber, finely sliced
1³/₄ oz. beansprouts
1 oz. watercress leaves (or baby spinach)
juice of half a lemon
2 tbsps fresh mint, chopped

1. Place the cucumber, sprouts, watercress leaves, and lemon juice in a bowl.
2. Pour over the lemon juice, sprinkle with fresh mint, and serve immediately.

8:30 p.m. Detox Bath
Use a few drops of the myrrh and frankincense oils in the bath. Remember not to make your bath too hot or too long. A 20-minute soak is just fine. Light some candles in the bathroom and relax.

Early to bed, early to rise makes you healthy, stealthy, and wise! Make sure that you get to bed early for maximum rest. Fill your hot water bottle with hot water. Lie down on your bed with the hot water bottle placed above your buttocks, in the lower and middle lower area of your back. You are essentially warming the kidneys and should feel pretty relaxed too. Also, remember to drink a cup of warm water an hour or so before bed.

24-Hour Detox Sachets
(OPTIONAL FOR A DEEPER CLEANSING)

After years of working with people suffering from toxicity
and weight issues, I developed a combination powder formula
for liver, gallbladder, and colon detox, available in health
foods shops. It works like a charm, and my clients swear by it.
It will give you one of the best clean-outs you have ever had.
But you will need to stay at home for 24 hours. My clients
call my 24-hour detox, "A colonic without a tube up the butt!"
It consists of pumpkin seeds, papayas, lemon
balm, magnesium, and oats.

DO YOU NEED ADRENAL CLEANSING?

Do you suffer from the following?

- ► Excess weight
- ► Beer belly or spare tire
- ► Middle Age spread or love handles
- ► Energy slumps mid-afternoon
- ► Difficulty getting out of bed
- ► Feeling constantly stressed

Poor adrenal function can hold back weight loss. It's important to give this gland a cleansing. My top tip is to take 15 drops of liquid Astragalus twice daily and a Vitamin B Complex, 50mg once a day for two months after the Detox. And for one month after that, take 15 drops of liquid Siberian Ginseng daily.

level four
slim for life

ASSESSMENT REPORT

At the very beginning of the book, I asked you to catalog a seven-day food and drink inventory. You collected all your food packaging for a week and analyzed the ingredients. You established your goals, banished your excuses, dumped your junk, and flicked the healthy eating switch. This was my way of setting you on the right path and giving you a starting point for your journey.

In life, it is important to take special moments to reflect on where you are. In other words, every so often it is helpful to look at the progress you are making. This process of reflection helps to motivate, inspire, encourage, foster hope, and also constructs a springboard from which you can leap to your next level. Now is that time. I want you to review and assess the progress that you have made since your starting point.

Following the guidelines within my plan, develop your own seven-day program. And while you follow your own plan, I want you to keep a diary of everything you eat and drink. After a week, compare your new diary with your original. I know you are going to see some amazing differences.

After that, I want you to complete the Self-Assessment Form.

Self-Assessment Form

1 What is the percentage of fresh food and vegetables in your diet now as opposed to before?

2 Are you now eating a greater variety of food groups and foods such as beans, whole grains, pulses, legumes, seeds, and seaweeds?

3 How much raw food are you eating now versus before?

4 Are you drinking more water?

5 How much healthier are your snacks compared with at the beginning?

6 Have you substantially reduced your intake of red meat, wheat, and milk products?

7 Have you drastically reduced or cut out the nasties—sugar, sweets, chocolate, caffeine, alcohol, and table salt?

8 How do you feel? Are you healthier?

9 Look in the mirror. What has changed about your body?

10 Do you have more energy now?

11 Is your digestion better?

12 Are you sleeping well?

13 Do you have more confidence preparing your own foods?

14 Are you exercising regularly?

15 Are you feeling happier, slimmer, and sexier?

HOW WOULD YOU RATE YOUR OVERALL GENERAL PROGRESS?

These are questions for you to ponder. I am not looking
for you to score anything. I just want you to reflect within
your own self by yourself.

EXCELLENT PROGRESS You are doing Fab!

GOOD PROGRESS Hang in there.

SATISFACTORY PROGRESS Could do better.

NO PROGRESS Back to the drawing board.

You need my SOS Emergency Plan (page 206).

THE 90/10 RULE

I have been called a stick in the mud, a party pooper, a food fascist, and the Diet Dictator! Yes, I am tough, and that's not going to change. I want you to get fantastic results. The bottom line is that I want you to get well and be healthier than you have ever been. I want you to reach your desired weight. And I know what it takes to get you there. It requires determination, willpower, drive, and a willingness to change.

During the plan I've owned you, but once you graduate you can move on to bigger and better things. After the eight weeks, I won't bop you over the head if you are compelled to deviate a tiny bit. Once you have proven yourself during my eight-week boot camp, I no longer require full 100 percent compliance. I call it my 90/10 Rule.

I used to tell my clients to use my 80/20 rule but I am now modifying that advice. Much to my chagrin, I have learned that some people are carefully working out how 20 percent of their meals can be bad. So I have decided to shift the percentages slightly, to 90/10. This way, there is less room for negative maneuvering.

It's Not about a Calculation

I am only talking figuratively. The 90/10 rule is nothing to do with numbers or calculations. Ultimately I want you to live the lifestyle 100 percent of the time, but I do also realize that at certain times, it may not be possible or desirable.

For example, you may go out for a date on a Saturday night and the restaurant has great desserts on offer and you want one of them. Go ahead and order it. Or you may have ordered a soup made with cream. It's okay to eat it. You may be on a long drive in the car where you have to stop at a motorway rest stop and they only have roasted nuts instead of raw. I don't want you to say, "Oh, I can't have that." The fact is, if you are hungry by all means go for the best of what you can get at that moment. It's okay because we have established that there is a figurative 90/10 rule. Do not feel guilty or beat yourself up over it because you now know that there is a guilt-free window of opportunity, albeit a small one.

What I don't want you to do is to calculate that 10 percent of your meals should be bad food. This would be the opposite of my intention. I would be horrified to think that you are trying to calculate bad food into your regimen. My intention is that you live a healthy lifestyle and do the best that you are able. So it's important to focus on the 90 percent.

Treats Can Be Goodies

Most people think that treats have to be bad for you. They have a point; most conventional treats are loaded with sugar, fat, and chemicals. Since childhood, we are conditioned to think that these treats taste good.

People are always terrified that there won't be any treats on my Plan. Not so. First, check out my *You Are What You Eat Cookbook* (Michael Joseph), which has full chapters on healthy and delicious treats, snacks, and quick bites.

I want you to change the mental association you might have with treats. As a child, you may have received sweets from parents, grandparents, aunts. Your brain makes an association with the taste of the treat and a feeling of love, giving, and happiness. It can leave an imprint for a lifetime, meaning that you then go after these treats to make you feel warm and loved again.

And to add insult to injury, sweets such as chocolate actually contain some ingredients that release feel-good chemicals in the brain. As a result, it is easy to fall into that treat trap.

If you think you might associate treats like cake and chocolate with feelings of happiness or comfort, then now is the perfect time to acknowledge it. You now know that foods laden with bad fats and refined sugars are far from good for you, so it's time to enjoy a whole new set of treats.

Treats That Won't Send You Back to Level One

Let me tell you a little story about treats. The other day
I was on the train to the airport. I sat next to a woman who was
delightedly chomping into a great big chocolate croissant with
a mountain of whipped cream on top. Totally oblivious to my
presence just inches away, she was savoring every crumb, but
just as she was about to indulge in her last bite, she casually
glanced around and caught my eye. She looked away, looked
nervously down at her crumbs, and then did a double take.

PASSENGER: Oh my God, it's you! I can't believe
you're sitting next to me in the train. I watch your show.
GILLIAN: So why did you eat that rubbish?
PASSENGER: I don't do this all the time.
GILLIAN: Was that your breakfast?
PASSENGER: Yes. But it was just a little treat.

I don't do, "Yes buts." I do, however, have lots of alternatives
to offer you. Treats do not need to be filled with sugar, chocolate,
wheat, additives, chemicals, and synthetic creams. When you
eat these kinds of foods, generally you are going to feel horrible
either right afterwards, shortly afterwards, or in the long-term.
It's a guarantee that you will affect your body negatively and
most likely feel it. Eat my healthy treats and you will feel good.
No guilt trip necessary.

GILLIAN'S ULTIMATE HEALTH TREATS

Sweet

- ► Fresh fruit such as grapes, strawberries, blueberries, and peaches
- ► Fruit salad
- ► Fruit smoothies
- ► Dried figs
- ► Prunes
- ► Medjool dates
- ► Natural organic yogurt, but it must be free of added sugar and sweeteners

Baked Apples (or Pears)

1. Preheat oven to 390°F.
2. Place 2 apples in an ovenproof dish.
3. Bake for 15–20 minutes.

Baked Figs with Agave and Lemon

SERVES 1
2 figs cut in half
1/2 tbsp agave syrup
juice of 1/2 lemon
1 star anise (optional)

1. Preheat the oven to 350°F.
2. Take a large piece of foil and place the halved figs in the center, pour over the syrup and lemon juice, and add the star anise if using.
3. Scrunch up the foil and place on a baking sheet.
Place in the oven and bake for 20 minutes.
4. Remove from the oven and allow to stand for 5 minutes.
Serve from the foil.

Strawberry Ice

For best results use an ice-cream maker. Alternatively, freeze in a shallow plastic container and whisk every 30 minutes with a fork until the mixture has frozen. It works well with raspberries too. Great treat for the kids.

MAKES 1 QUART
18 oz. fresh hulled strawberries plus extra to garnish
2 tbsps agave syrup
2 cups rice milk
mint leaves to garnish

1. Place the strawberries in the food processor or blender and blend until smooth. Add the agave syrup and rice milk and blend for a further 30 seconds.
2. Pour into an ice-cream maker and leave to churn for 20 to 30 minutes.
3. Scoop into a glass dish and garnish with fresh fruit and mint leaves.

Mango Granita

This healthy reward will keep well in the freezer for up to a month, so it is worth making a batch when mangoes are ripe and inexpensive. Allow to thaw for 5 to 10 minutes at room temperature before serving.

2 ripe mangoes
juice of 1 lime
$1/2$ cup cold water
4 bunches fresh red currants

1. With a sharp knife cut the cheeks from the sides of the mangoes. Cut these in half and then slide the knife blade under the skin to remove the flesh. Trim as much flesh from the pit as possible and place all of it in the food processor or blender.
2. Blend until you have a smooth pulp. Add the lime juice and water and process for 15 more seconds.
3. Pour the puree into a plastic container and place in the freezer.
4. Every 30 minutes whisk the mixture vigorously with a fork. The sorbet should be ready in 2–3 hours and should appear quite grainy in texture.
5. Serve in tall-stemmed glasses garnished with fresh red currants or other fruit.

Rhubarb Crumble

When cooking fruits such as rhubarb, do not allow the fruit to boil. It should simply cook at a low simmer. This will ensure that as many of the nutrients as possible are preserved. Rhubarb is an excellent source of calcium.

SERVES 2
3¹/₂ oz. rhubarb, chopped
¹/₂ tbsp agave syrup
¹/₃ cup cold water
FOR THE TOPPING
1³/₄ oz. oats
¹/₂ tbsp millet flour
1 tbsp agave syrup

1. Place the rhubarb, agave syrup, and water in a small pan. Cook over a gentle heat for 15 minutes. Remove from the heat, allow to cool slightly, and then transfer to a small pie dish.
2. Preheat the oven to 350°F.
3. Place the oats and flour in a mixing bowl and stir well. Then mix in the syrup. The mixture will appear a little lumpy.
4. Scatter the mixture over the fruit. Do not press the mixture down.
5. Transfer to the oven and bake for 15 minutes until the top is crisp.
6. Remove from the oven and allow to stand for 5 minutes before serving.

Date and Almond Truffles

8 fresh dates
3¹/₂ oz. ground almonds
2 tsps carob powder
finely grated rind and freshly squeezed juice of lime
macadamia nuts or Brazil nuts (optional)
chopped mixed nuts (optional)

1. Place the dates, almonds, carob powder,
lime rind, and juice into a food processor.
2. Blend until the mixture forms a stiff ball.
3. Add more lime juice if necessary to help bring
the mixture together.
4. Remove blade and roll date mixture into balls.
Place in truffle cases or roll in chopped, mixed nuts.
5. Fill each with a macadamia or Brazil nut.
6. Cover and keep in the fridge.

Lemon Tofu Chiffon Cake

12 oz. pack firm silken tofu
3 tbsps agave syrup
rind of 2 lemons plus juice of 2
3½ oz. gram or chickpea flour
2 tsps baking powder
2 tbsps water

1. Preheat the oven to 340°F. Line a small loaf pan, approximately 8" by 4", with baking parchment.
2. Place the tofu, syrup, lemon rind, and juice in a mixing bowl and beat with an electric mixer until smooth and light. This will take 5 minutes.
3. Mix the baking powder and flour together and beat into the tofu 2 tbsps at a time. Whisk with the mixer for an additional 5 minutes.
4. Transfer to the prepared tin and bake for 25–30 minutes until firm but still springy to the touch. Remove from the oven and allow to cool slightly and then lift out with the baking parchment and allow to cool completely.
5. Serve in slices.

Carrot Cake

Agave syrup happens to taste sweet and comes from
the cactus plant.

3½ oz. grated carrot
2 oranges
4 tbsps agave syrup
1 free-range egg
5¼ oz. gram or chickpea flour
½ tsp baking powder
3½ oz. soft silken tofu

1. Preheat the oven to 340°F. Line a small loaf pan with
baking parchment.
2. Grate the orange zest. Place the carrot, zest of 1½ oranges,
and half the syrup in a mixing bowl. Stir with a fork and make
a hole in the center.
3. Break the egg into the hole and whisk the egg until light
and frothy.
4. Mix the flour with the baking powder and then beat into
the carrot mixture 2 tablespoonfuls at a time.
5. Add the juice of 1 orange and mix well. Place half the juice
of the second orange in the base of the loaf pan.
6. Transfer the carrot mixture to the prepared pan and smooth
the surface with a pallet knife. Place in the preheated oven and
bake for 25–30 minutes or until well risen, golden in color, and
firm to the touch.
7. Remove from the oven and lift the cake out of the pan using
the parchment. Allow to cool.
8. Beat the tofu with the remaining syrup until light and
smooth, then add the juice of half an orange. Stir well to mix
and leave to stand for a few minutes.
9. When the cake is cold, top with the frosting, sprinkle over
the remaining zest, and serve.

Vanilla and Cinnamon Rice Pudding

SERVES 1
1¹/₂ cups water or rice milk
3¹/₂ oz. organic short grain brown rice
¹/₄ stick cinnamon
¹/₄ vanilla pod
zest and juice of ¹/₂ orange
1 tbsp agave syrup (if you use rice milk,
you won't need the agave)

1. Place the water or rice milk in a small saucepan, add the rice, cinnamon, vanilla, orange zest and juice, and the syrup if using.
2. Bring to a boil, cover, and simmer for 25–30 minutes, stirring occasionally.

Carob Mousse

SERVES 4
4 tsps carob powder
4 tsps very hot water
8$\frac{1}{2}$ oz. soft silken tofu
4 tsps rice syrup
4 tsps agave syrup
6 drops pure vanilla essence
freshly ground cinnamon to taste
4 sprigs of mint to garnish

1. Place the carob in a small bowl, add the hot water, and mix well until the carob powder has dissolved.
2. Place the tofu in a medium-sized bowl and whisk with a balloon whisk or electric whisk until it is smooth.
3. Beat the liquid carob mixture into the tofu, then beat in the rice syrup followed by the agave syrup. Whisk well between each addition.
4. Add the vanilla essence and cinnamon, whisk just to combine, then transfer to four small glasses or glass dishes.
5. Chill for 30 minutes or up to 2 hours. Serve garnished with a sprig of mint.

Savory

- **Vegetable juices**
- **Oatcakes**
- **Rice cakes with mashed avocado, hummus, and dill—topped off with tomato halves**
- **Vegetable crudités with hummus or other healthy dips (see page 200)**
- **Soaked almonds or soaked nuts of any sort (soaking nuts overnight always makes them easier to digest and sweeter tasting)**
- **Nuts**
- **Steamed nuts**
- **Raw shelled hemp seeds mashed into avocados**
- **Raw shelled hemp seeds with anything!**
- **Roasted sweet potatoes with mashed avocados and herbs such as basil**
- **Shitake mushrooms on wheat-free toast**
- **Sautéed pumpkin seeds with wheat-free tamari sauce**

Baked Beets

Preheat oven to 390°F
Wrap in foil and bake for 30 minutes

Baked Sweet Potatoes

Preheat oven to 390°F
Wrap in foil and bake for 30 minutes

Baked and Sliced Butternut Squash

Preheat oven to 390°F
Wrap in foil and bake for 45 minutes

Baked Yams

Preheat oven to 390°F
Wrap in foil and bake for 30 minutes

Calzones with Cherry Tomatoes and Zucchini

If it's pizza that you miss, then try these. You need to take a little care with the pastry or it will break up. If it does, don't worry too much, just press it back together.

MAKES 4
9 3/4 oz. cherry tomatoes, halved
1 bunch scallions, finely chopped
1 tbsp water (for tomato sauce)
2 tbsps freshly chopped basil
1 tbsp fresh oregano
7 oz. buckwheat flour
2 tsps baking powder
2 tsps olive oil
2/3 cup water (for pastry)
3 1/2 oz. zucchini cut into 1/2" slices
fresh arugula to garnish

1. Place the cherry tomatoes, scallions, and water in a small pan and simmer gently over a low heat for 5–6 minutes. Remove from the heat and allow to cool, then mix in the herbs.
2. Preheat the oven to 390°F.
3. Mix the flour and baking powder in a bowl. Make a hole in the center, add the oil and 1/2 cup of the water. Mix gently, adding more water as required to make a soft dough.
4. Knead gently on a floured clean surface and divide the dough into four pieces and roll them out to form circles.
5. Divide the tomato mixture between the dough circles and top with the zucchini slices. Carefully fold the dough over to form half-moon shapes.
6. Transfer to a baking pan lined with parchment paper and bake for 10–12 minutes.
7. Remove from the oven and allow to cool for 5 minutes, before serving with the arugula garnish.

Dips

Spinach Dip

1 avocado, peeled with pit removed
juice of $\frac{1}{2}$ lemon
8 oz.-can organic chickpeas, drained
7 oz. fresh spinach

1. Place the avocado in the bowl of the processor with the lemon juice and chickpeas and process until you have a smooth paste.
2. Place the spinach in a steamer and steam for 1–2 minutes until just wilted. Remove from the heat and allow to cool slightly. Drain, then squeeze the spinach with your hand or the back of a spoon to remove any excess liquid.
3. Add the spinach to the avocado and chickpeas and process for a few seconds to combine. Transfer to a bowl and serve.

Cucumber and Garlic Dip

12 oz. pack soft tofu
3–4 cloves garlic, peeled
handful of fresh mint leaves
$\frac{1}{4}$ cucumber, finely diced
lemon juice to taste

1. Place the tofu in the bowl of the food processor and process until smooth.
2. With the motor running add the garlic and then the mint leaves.
3. Transfer the mixture to a bowl and stir in the cucumber and some lemon juice to taste.
4. Serve immediately.

Minted Eggplant Dip

1 small eggplant
2 plump garlic cloves
3 tbsps extra virgin olive oil
2 tbsps freshly squeezed lemon juice
2 tbsps chopped fresh mint
¹/₂ tsp ground cumin

1. Preheat the oven to 390°F.
2. Halve the eggplant. Peel the garlic and cut each clove into 4–5 slices.
3. Make a few deep incisions into the cut side of each eggplant half and place a slice of garlic well into each one.
4. Place eggplant halves on a baking tray and drizzle with 1 tbsp of the olive oil. Bake, cut side up, for 35–45 minutes until very tender and pale golden brown.
5. Remove from the oven and leave for about 20 minutes until cool enough to handle.
6. Using a dessertspoon, scoop the eggplant center and softened garlic into a food processor, discarding the skin. Add the remaining olive oil, lemon juice, mint, and cumin. Blend until smooth.

Inedible Treats

Treat yourself in different ways too. Try these ideas or create your own luxury moments.

- **A sauna**
- **A swim**
- **A massage**
- **A facial**
- **A reflexology session**
- **Find a quiet space for meditation**
- **Watch a film**
- **Buy a new CD or DVD**
- **Treat yourself to a new outfit**
- **Read a good novel**
- **Take up a new hobby like tennis, racketball, tai chi, kickboxing, dancing, karate, ice skating, or whatever tickles your fancy**

A Quick Guide to Eating Out

The first rule of eating out is to enjoy yourself. If you eat out regularly, then you do need to be more careful, but if it's an occasional treat, then I wouldn't want you to feel guilt over the salad dressing on the way home.

In restaurants, don't take it to extremes, and don't try to force others to make the same choices as you. You want to be able to enjoy your time out, and so do your dining partners. Here are a few guidelines to help keep eating out healthy, delicious, and enjoyable:

- Don't starve yourself in anticipation of a restaurant meal. You are not on a calorie-controlled diet.

- Twenty minutes before you eat, drink a glass of still water with no ice. You'll feel fuller and will digest the meal better. You can have little sips of water during the meal but no beer or carbonated drinks.

- Order first, so you won't be tempted or swayed by other people's (possibly unhealthy) choices. You may even set the stage for healthy eating for all.

- Order a vegetarian-based soup for starters, if possible. Try to avoid the dairy cream-based soups, and ask that cream not be added. Most soups will fill you up and are easy to digest. They are a great wholesome choice when eating out.

- Stop eating when you are two-thirds full. Listen to the cues your body gives you. It takes a while for your stomach's messages to get through to the brain, hence that overstuffed feeling you might get. You don't have to leave your plate empty. Ask how dishes are prepared. Waiters are becoming accustomed to these types of questions, so don't worry about asking. Here are some of the questions you might want to pose:

  - Are your dishes baked? (good)

  - Are they grilled? (good)

  - Are they prepared with butter? (bad) Or oil? (fine if not fried)

  - Is the fish wild? (good) Or farmed? (bad)

Ask what's in the sauce; ask what's in the soup; ask what's in the dressing. Excessive sugar and too much salt is what you are trying to avoid.

- Take your time. Put your knife and fork down between each bite. Take no notice of how quickly others may be eating.

- You can ask for the gravy, sauce, or salad dressing to be served on the side. That way, if you don't like it or it comes laden with butter or sugar, it has not spoiled your meal. You can always ask for a lemon to squeeze over your fish or salad instead. But don't worry too much if the sauce or dressing is an integral part of the dish.

- Feel free to order two starters, or a starter and then a salad or combination of side dishes—not including fries! For example, I might have an artichoke heart salad to start and a combination of green beans, spinach, and almond rice as my main course.

- If you are going out to a Chinese, Japanese, or Thai restaurant, make sure they do not use MSG (monosodium glutamate) in their dishes.

► If you are ordering pasta, go for a tomato-based sauce rather than a cream-based sauce. Simpler dishes are often the most delicious.

► Order off-menu if you have to. You could ask for grilled fish with vegetables and a salad made with oil and no butter. Or you could ask the chef what he/she can do for a vegetarian/vegan meal. Can he create something that is meat and dairy free? What can he come up with?

► If you're thinking about dessert, wait about 10 minutes after finishing your main meal before ordering. Give your stomach time to tell your brain if it has had enough. If you still can't resist the chocolate delight, you can always split the dessert with your dining partner and let them eat the lion's share. Often a few bites are enough to satisfy.

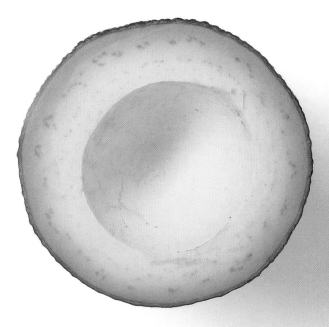

Dr. Gillian's SOS Emergency Plan

If you've noticed yourself wandering off the path a few
too many times, then you may need a jump start. After all,
you don't want to go hurtling back to Level One.

DAY 1

If you have gone off the rails, don't fret. The last thing
I want you to feel is that it's game over and that you might as
well slip all the way down the slope and forget about healthy
eating altogether. It's easy to come back. Every day is a brand
new day where you can start again. And most important of
all, YOU ARE NOT ON A DIET. So you cannot fall off the diet,
fall off the wagon, or eat too many calories. There's nothing
to fall off. When you picked up this book, it was to embark on
a lifestyle change. That is a completely different concept from
going on a diet. As one person put it on my website forum,
"Gillian's way is a state of mind. It is not a diet and therefore
not something that you can stop."

I do demand that you embrace this healthy lifestyle as wholly
as you can and commit to it 100 percent. But if something crazy
happens in your life and you veer off, so what? Don't worry about
it. Just keep doing what you set out to do. Keep embracing
the lifestyle. So if last Monday you missed breakfast and ate
a croissant in the middle of the day, you have not failed.

- ▶ **Acknowledge it**
- ▶ **Recognize it**
- ▶ **Take note of it**
- ▶ **Use it as a marker to stay on the path**

On Day 1 of your SOS Plan, the party you were invited to is canceled. The after-work-drinks-meeting is postponed. I need your focus, effort, and resolve.

Drink a cup of warm water with a squeeze of lemon right now. Then make sure that you drink another cup one hour before bed. Drink eight cups of warm water and plenty of herbal teas during the next three days. To get it all in, one rule of thumb is to drink one glass per hour. The only two teas I want you to drink today are nettle or dandelion. Take your pick. No moaning. I don't want to hear it.

Photocopy the SOS Emergency Exercise. You are going to use this for the next three days. Carry it with you wherever you go. Every two hours you will need to conduct the Emergency Exercise. It does not matter where you are, you could be on the plane, train, bus, at your desk in the office, in the kitchen, wherever.

Dr. Gillian's SOS Emergency Exercise

1. Close your eyes.
2. Listen to your breath.
3. Count up from 1 to 10.
4. Repeat slowly the following words 10 times, to yourself silently, or aloud. "I live my new Lifestyle for life."
5. At the end of the 10 repetitions, visualize a movie screen with you in the lead role. In this film, you view a full day of your life acting out the lifestyle. So, for example, you see yourself eating a healthy breakfast; you witness yourself doing a 20-minute walk before a meal; you eat a fabulously healthy lunch; and so on. At the end of the day in the movie, you see yourself happy, content, and harmonized. And you are fully on track.
6. Count back down from 10 to 1.
7. Slowly open your eyes.

Day 1

DATE:

MANTRA

Write the following statement 10 times: **I promise to eat breakfast.**

_____

_____

_____

_____

_____

_____

_____

_____

_____

_____

BREAKFAST

Go out to your local supermarket and buy a large fresh fruit salad already prepared or make your own. That will be your breakfast. Easy.

Chop up some raw fresh vegetables or buy them already pre-chopped from a supermarket. Get a selection of cucumbers, carrots, red or yellow peppers, endive, and snow peas. Take them to work and eat them before, during, and after lunch as snacks. You can dip them in hummus.

LUNCH

Miso Soup. That's what you are having. Buy it from a health food store. Pour the packet into a mug and add hot water. Have two mugs of miso soup.

AFTER WORK

Go home, turn on the radio to your favorite station, and dance like crazy. Jump up and down, yell, sing out loud. But most important, get moving. (See page 74 for other exercise ideas.)

DINNER

After exercise, you must have a vegetable juice and follow it with a crunchy salad with sauerkraut and lemon squeezed over. If you live near a place that makes fresh vegetable juices, go and buy the juice. If not, make it yourself. It will take five minutes and is well worth the small effort.

SOS Juice

4 carrots
¹/₂ apple
2 celery sticks
1 cucumber
tiny piece of ginger

Get to bed by 10:00 p.m. for the next three days.

So you got through Day 1. Well done. Now it's on to Day 2.

Plan your exact food menu in advance for the next day. I have given you space below to do this. To make it even easier for you, all you have to do is choose from the list provided on page 212. Advance planning is critical to staying onboard. You will notice that much of the food is raw/uncooked, so preparation is minimal.

Day 2

MANTRA
Write out the following statement 10 times: **I am on track with Gillian.**

BREAKFAST

SNACK

SNACK

DINNER

LUNCH

EXERCISE

Day 3

DATE:

MANTRA

Write out the following statement 10 times: **I am on track, and I promise to eat breakfast.**

BREAKFAST

SNACK

SNACK

DINNER

LUNCH

EXERCISE

BREAKFAST CHOICES

Start each day with one cup of warm water with a squeeze of lemon juice, followed by a cup of nettle tea, then choose from:

Apple/pear/peach/pineapple salad
2 pink grapefruit

Strawberry Banana Smoothie
Simply blend one small basket of strawberries, one ripe banana, and a 1/2 cup water until smooth.

Millet Oatmeal
It's comforting and creamy and tastes like oatmeal but with a fluffy, soothing texture.

1 3/4 oz. millet flakes
1 3/4 oz. oat flakes
1 2/3 cups water

1. Bring the millet, oats, and water to a boil in a pan.
2. Lower the heat and simmer for 3–5 minutes, stirring until you get the desired consistency. Sprinkle with dried herbs or a pinch of sea salt and serve.

It only takes minutes, so no excuses now.

SNACKS FOR MID-MORNING

Choose from the following:
Apple
Pear
Grapes
Pineapple juice
Pink grapefruit juice
Vegetable juice. Either make your own and take it with you in a flask or buy one that is organic with no added sugar.

SNACKS FOR MID-AFTERNOON

Choose from the following:
At least a cup or more of crunchy sugar snap peas
Handful of raw, unsalted Brazil nuts
Vitality Juice (page 173)

LUNCH CHOICES

Miso Soup with Tofu
Chop a small slab of tofu into bite-sized cubes and throw into the soup.

Any kind of bean, vegetable, or miso soup (either make your own or buy a sugar free veggie soup).
Follow the soup with a crunchy, green leafy salad.

DINNER

Appetizer: MUST HAVE vegetable juice
1 whole baby gem lettuce
6 celery stalks
1 fennel
1 cucumber
1 apple (optional for sweetness)

Baked Sweet Potato with Avocado and Warm Vegetable Salad

Get your taste buds ready for a hot baked sweet potato with a kick of cumin to satisfy any little cravings, buttery sliced avocado, fresh peppery leaves, and warm vegetables—my ultimate feel-good foods.

SERVES 1
1 medium sweet potato—around 9 oz.
½ yellow pepper
4 cherry tomatoes
1 tsp olive oil
2 large handfuls wild arugula leaves
½ ripe avocado
cress (optional)
ground cumin to taste
DRESSING
1 tbsp olive oil
1 tsp organic balsamic vinegar
½ crushed clove garlic

1. Wash the potato and dry with kitchen paper. Place on a baking tray and cook in a preheated oven at 390°F for about 40 minutes until tender.
2. Thinly slice the yellow pepper and cut the cherry tomatoes in half.
3. Remove the tray from the oven and add the pepper and tomatoes. Drizzle with 1 tsp olive oil and return to the oven for 5 minutes.
4. Place the wild arugula leaves in a bowl and top with the sliced ripe avocado. Snip a little cress—if you have some handy—and sprinkle on top. Remove the potato and vegetables from the oven.
5. Place the potato on a plate, split it open, and sprinkle with a good pinch of ground cumin. Scatter the warmed pepper and tomatoes over the salad. Toss together very lightly. Drizzle with 1 tbsp olive oil and 1 tsp organic balsamic vinegar mixed with half a crushed garlic clove. Serve with the hot potato.

EASY DINNER OPTIONS

1. Baked beans on wheat-free toast. Health food stores carry sugar free and sweetener free versions of baked beans. Serve with parsnip mash. Boil parsnips and mash with a little olive oil. If you can't get parsnips, use rutabaga, turnips, yams, or squash. Add some baby gem lettuce and sprinkle with torn basil and chopped cilantro.
2. Wheat-free pasta from a health food store or supermarket. Purchase an organic sugar-free sauce for pasta. Health food stores carry tomato-free sauces too. Toss with torn fresh basil leaves.
3. Tray of grilled veggies on a bed of green leaves. Slice and place a beet, a parsnip, onion, peppers, eggplant, or zucchini on a tray and drizzle with oil and a sprinkling of dried herbs. Simply grill and serve with fresh salad leaves and fresh basil.

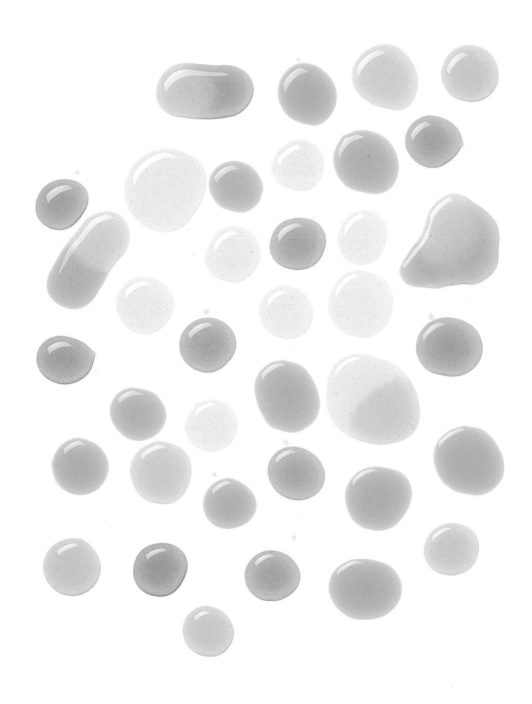

WHY MY SOS EMERGENCY PLAN WORKS

This mini plan I have devised is simple and uncomplicated.
It's enough for you to stay on track, while also addressing
your comfort needs. It's all of the following:

- **Easy**
- **Comforting**
- **Quick**
- **Fulfilling (you will not feel hungry)**
- **Inexpensive**
- **Uncomplicated**
- **A cinch**
- **Something to look forward to**
- **Enjoyable**
- **Focused**

You will feel better almost immediately on two levels: physically
and mentally. You are treating your body with the respect that
it deserves and you have taken definitive, positive steps. You will
now have the incentive to keep going over the long term, and you
should notice that you have more energy, are less bloated, and
have the motivation to carry on with the lifestyle. You have not
fallen by the wayside. You are on track. The sky is the limit
with the results you can achieve.

Dr. Gillian's Final Word for Ultimate Health

So now you know what to do. You have the tools for ultimate health. If you follow my plan, there are no failures. I truly hope that I have turned you on to the amazing possibilities that simple changes in eating and lifestyle can bring. I want you to feel fabulous now and for life. Here are some final words of advice I want to share with you . . .

Point One You need to care about what goes into your mouth. What you put in is what you will get out. Put in good food, and you will feel the benefits. Food is energy, so fill up on the good stuff. Think about how well your body will run on pure, natural foods versus artificial foods empty of any real nutrition, taste, or energy.

Point Two Food is one type of energy; your thoughts are also crucial points of energy. Keep your thoughts pure and positive. Like the food you eat, what you put into your head also affects your whole makeup. Fill yourself with happy thoughts and you will feel and be happier.

Point Three Your emotions are the window to your body and soul. I want you to take stock of your emotions every day. How do you feel today? Your emotions are your antennae to your inner alignment. Your emotions will tell you if your thoughts are properly aligned with your feelings. If your thoughts are taking you in the right direction that's best suited for you, then your emotions will feel positive. Conversely, if your thoughts are moving in a direction that is not right for you, then your emotional antennae will let you know by the way that you feel. Listen to your heart.

Point Four Be confident with the new you. You need not act out life based on what someone else tells you to do, or what you think you should do, or what some institution commands is right for you. The "shoulds" and the "oughts" are fantasy. Listening to the dictates of others only displaces your alignment with your thoughts and feelings. There is only one way to know what is best for you and how to act: Look within and feel your inner thoughts and emotions. Feel your soul, your inner core. Listen to the deepest you. Then you will know what is right for you, how to think, and when to act.

Let me share a story of my own with you. Not too long ago, I was scheduled to take a trip abroad. I thought that I had to go. It was all planned. Other people were counting on me to show up. And even my own head said, "You've got to go there." But in a very quiet moment of stillness, I knew in my gut that it did not feel right. I even said to a colleague, "I know that I should take this trip, but in my belly I feel it will be wrong."

So my thoughts and feelings were not aligned. I was out of sync with myself. Worse yet, I ignored my feeling of not wanting to go. As it turned out, this would prove to be a nightmarish trip. On every level, from the terrible airplane ride to horrific weather conditions to scheduling mishaps, everything went wrong, and not just for the one day but for all four days.

Point Five You attract in life the very same vibrations that you personally vibrate. Give out good energy and you will attract good energy. If you vibrate energies of sadness, anger, fear, disappointment, frustration, blame, resentment, and the like, then you will attract these same negative energies toward you. Negative energy can manifest in all shapes, sizes, and forms, and I have discovered in practice that when people emit negative energy, they will be far more likely to make poor food choices. And conversely, when you are feeling happy and thinking positively, you will be more prone to making the right healthy food choices. Furthermore, when you eat healthy foods, you are likely to feel and think in a more positive and clear way. Happy thoughts attract good food choices and vice versa—the perfect cycle of Ultimate Health.

Point Six Every day (and actually every moment of life) is a new day and a new moment for you to re-create yourself. In other words, just because you had negative thoughts yesterday doesn't mean that you need them today. Or if your thoughts were out of sync with your feelings earlier today, then in the evening you can still choose to get back into harmony. For instance, you have a fight with your partner before you both leave for work. You know that you still feel intense love for each other. When you both return home, you decide to kiss and make up. You have made a conscious choice here to change the energy between the two of you via the thought and actions of resolution. You can use this application in any aspect of your life. You can literally switch on positive or switch off negative thoughts if you make a conscious decision to do so.

Point Seven The bottom line here is that you can change your life. You can make choices and eliminate resistance. You get to decide: good food, positive lifestyle, wellness, great body, slim figure, unconditional love, joy, fulfillment, happiness . . . ultimate health. It's all in your hands.

Wishing you Love & Light,

Gillian

Index

Dear Dad: This book is dedicated to you, Dad. Miss you so much. But I feel you close and know you are watching over. Your signs have reaffirmed for me that there is more to life than what we can see, feel, think, touch, and smell.

Squeezes, hugs, kisses, cuddles, and love to my two wee lassies. You are so loved and cherished. And to my immense, outstanding foundation and inspiration, Howard: You are a gifted catalyst for transformation of the planet on so many levels. Your motivation, huge support, passion, words, and contributions are life-altering and deeply appreciated.

I wish to thank every person who has opened one of my books, flicked on the switch to watch the *You Are What You Eat* television series or written me a letter of blessing. It is each and every one of you who are making it possible to get my message out to the world.

Enormous gratitude, thanks, and love to my editor, Kate Adams. You are an exceptional person whose heart and soul is also in this book. Your commitment is inspiring. And to everyone at Smith & Gilmour. Thank you for your tremendous hard work—your design is superb and your creativity unmatched. And thank you to all at Penguin, particularly Tom Weldon, Louise Moore, and Sarah Rollason.

Deep appreciation to Helen T. Big hugs to your kids and hubby too. We know our grams inside out now.

Nicola, you are so special and along with Julia, Jo, Dawn, Johnny, Gina, and Helen you are a tremendous team. You all hold a warm place in my heart. THANK YOU for everything. And dearest Luigi: You are an absolute gem.

To my wonderful Max Clifford, much love. Your guidance and kindness is unsurpassed. And to the fantastic Lucy, Louise, Jessica, and all at MCA. You are doing wonders.

Big thanks to Theresa for your in-depth research. And to Josie for your excellent support.

Justine. You are a fabulous creative mind.

Thanks to Zdrafka and Izabela for keeping it all together and trying out recipe after recipe. Adzuki Bean Bake. It rocks!

Oscar, you are still getting me from A to B on time, even when I am not. And dispensing words of wisdom in the process.

To my rocks, Doug and Eloise, a big hug. Gratitude to George, Paul, David, Placy, Leonora, and the gang.

To my pillars of strength at McKeith Research Ltd: Nonedible treats take on a whole new meaning with you, Alan. You are an incredible individual. Alan, Rob, Indranie, and Jon: You are spearheading a movement of enormous change. You are all always there for me, towers of strength. Words don't do justice to how much I am grateful for all that you do.

Chaim Solomon: You get me through and keep me on my spiritual path. You are remarkable.

Much love to Mum. Your encouragement keeps me going strong.

www.drgillianmckeith.com

The Dr. Gillian McKeith website is designed to be the ultimate source for active support, help, and information. It brings the whole Dr. Gillian philosophy to life.

Come on over to the website and discover slimming support, diet help, nutritional information, allergy testing, resource guides, the McKeith Research Centre, free e-newsletters, Live Chat, the Dr. Gillian Website Club, and a one-stop shop.